The Acupuncture Points Functions Colouring Book

THE Acupuncture
POINTS FUNCTIONS
COLOURING BOOK

Rainy Hutchinson

Forewords by Angela Hicks and John Hicks, and Richard Blackwell

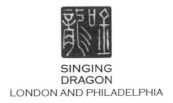

SINGING
DRAGON
LONDON AND PHILADELPHIA

The points functions text is reproduced with kind permission from the College of Integrated Chinese Medicine.

First published in 2015
by Singing Dragon
an imprint of Jessica Kingsley Publishers
73 Collier Street
London N1 9BE, UK
and
400 Market Street, Suite 400
Philadelphia, PA 19106, USA

www.singingdragon.com

Library of Congress Cataloging in Publication Data
A CIP catalog record for this book is available from the Library of Congress

British Library Cataloguing in Publication Data
A CIP catalogue record for this book is available from the British Library

ISBN 978 1 84819 266 9
eISBN 978 0 85701 214 2

Printed and bound in Great Britain

Contents

Foreword

Rainy qualified from the College of Integrated Chinese Medicine in 2003. From the beginning of the course she used her drawing skills as a learning tool to help her to remember acupuncture points. We enjoyed watching her combining her artistic talents with her study and using the metaphors of the point names to form memorable pictures. We still have one of her pictures hanging on the wall in the college building. The picture stands out and is much admired by many people who see it.

It is now well-documented that everyone has a preferred learning style. These roughly divide into four categories – visual, kinaesthetic, tactile and auditory. At the College of Integrated Chinese Medicine the students are shown ways to discover which ones they prefer. Knowing this enables them to use their favoured learning style to their advantage when they study.

In China students put the theory of Chinese medicine into rhymes and recite them as a way of remembering. Learning point locations, pulse diagnosis and other practical techniques is often a more kinaesthetic or tactile way of learning. The point names, however, are usually best learnt visually. Names such as 'eyes bright', 'blazing valley' and 'sun and moon', for example, conjure up images that can be instantly remembered.

There is now a large body of evidence to show how much the visual mode helps us to remember information. This makes sense when we consider that our brains are mainly 'image processors' rather than 'word processors'. In fact, the part of the brain used to process words is quite small compared with the part used to process visual images.

As soon as students make visual associations their recall of information is much better than if they merely read through their notes or try to remember the words. We live in a visual society and from an early age this is our main mode of learning. For this reason many people find their learning style preferences have some leaning towards the visual mode.

We are delighted to support Rainy in her work of putting these pictures into a book for others to enjoy. They take us on a journey and enable us to travel through the point names and functions to make them easily memorable.

This book can be used by students and practitioners alike and may also be of interest to patients and members of the public who enjoy knowing about the names of the acupuncture points.

Rainy is both a talented practitioner and a talented artist. The combination of her talents comes together in this delightful colouring book and we hope it helps many others to learn the point names.

Angela Hicks and John Hicks
Joint Principals and Co-Founders,
The College of Integrated Chinese Medicine

Foreword

It is hard work, being an acupuncture student. The challenges students face include gaining an in-depth understanding of a whole approach to medicine that is rooted in two millennia of Chinese culture and language and recorded in libraries full of clinical information. At the same time they are learning a substantial amount of biomedicine and mastering all the other skills and knowledge that contribute to the process of becoming a professional healthcare practitioner. In the midst of all this, students often say that learning the functions (or actions) of the acupuncture points is a particular challenge. Students find that they need as many aids to their learning as possible, and this book is a helpful addition to the aids available to them.

Learning about the functions of the acupuncture points requires a certain amount of rote learning. Unfortunately, rote learning has been rather devalued in modern education and is sometimes spoken of somewhat dismissively as 'surface learning'. However, it is clearly important in clinical practice to have this sort of information available for instant recall. A more traditional approach would see the initial rote learning as a pre-condition for the gradual development of a much deeper understanding that one sees in experienced practitioners. This is supported from the perspective of our developing understanding of neuro-plasticity,

the science behind the remarkably flexible ways in which our brains change as we learn, in which rote learning is a way of reinforcing new connections in our minds that help to create the foundations for new ways of thinking and perceiving.

In education, much has been made of a range of ideas about learning styles. In their early days of studying for their degree, undergraduates are often encouraged to complete questionnaires designed to help them to understand their own personal learning style, their preferred way of learning. For example, one popular categorisation from Neil Fleming is into visual, auditory, reading-writing and kinaesthetic/tactile learning styles. Just how much difference it makes to students' outcomes when teachers apply these ideas is now contested, but many students say they find it helpful to learn more about themselves in this way and to apply these ideas to the way they study. The truth of the matter may well be that most of us learn best by using as many of our senses as possible. This means that this book's highly visual approach to the functions of key acupuncture points will be of value to many acupuncture students, nicely complementing the more linear text-based approach found in most of their books, and the verbal input from their tutors. Even better, this is a book to interact with and for many the tactile experience of colouring the graphics

and even adding one's own notes will greatly assist the learning process. Further value is added because at the same time as learning the functions of the points, students are also learning the pathways of all the main channels. In addition there is good use of cartoons and visual mnemonics, both of which have long been used to help information to lodge securely in memory.

Learning the functions of the acupuncture points is important and valuable, but also challenging. At the heart of all good medicine is the art of choosing the best treatment for each patient, based on a diagnosis that is specific to them as an individual. The functions of the acupuncture points are a way of codifying the experience of generation after generation of acupuncturists in China, capturing both broad principles and specific details to assist practitioners in making their choice of best treatment. This book will help the practitioners of the future to absorb more easily this therapeutically valuable information, and hence ultimately to achieve the best outcomes for their patients, and that is all most welcome.

Richard Blackwell
Principal, Northern College of Acupuncture

Acknowledgements

I would like to thank the College of Integrated Chinese Medicine in Reading UK for allowing me to use their text in the making of this book. Since all of the drawings were based directly on this text while I was a student at the college, I am most grateful to be able to reproduce them here. I am also indebted to Angela and John Hicks for their kind help and support over the course of this project.

Without the numerous prompts and words of encouragement from my dear friend and colleague Yvonne Sommer, I would never have got started on this book, the components of which lay dormant in a box under my bed for 13 years. She convinced me that the positive feedback from fellow students regarding the drawings had not been simple politeness but a genuine indication of wider appeal.

I am extremely grateful to Claire Wilson from Singing Dragon for her enthusiasm and patient guidance through all the twists and turns of bringing this project to completion. Thanks also to my cousin Molly Ruttan-Moffat in Los Angeles for her help in preparing the early original drawings for print, and to my family, especially my husband Mark for his support throughout.

Rainy Hutchinson
2015

Introduction

The Acupuncture Points Functions Colouring Book is intended as a learning tool, an aide-mémoire for students of acupuncture. It attempts to provide a map of the channels so that an overview of each channel can be gained and revised at a glance. The maps flow around their page in sequence as energy flows through the meridians. Each map offers a sense of the whole channel, as well as a sense of the nature of individual points. It is intended that these drawings should provide a framework for further learning and study. The book is designed to be flexible enough to accommodate the needs of students from a wide range of schools and disciplines, as it must be recognised that, within the traditions of Chinese Medicine, different colleges have different approaches to the learning of this information.

Some colleges emphasise certain functions above others; some always link the teaching of point functions with point location. Some highlight element points, while others give only passing reference to these. Point names also vary widely from one school to another. These variations are all the inevitable result of a rich heritage that has developed and evolved over thousands of years.

It should be remembered that, by necessity, these drawings are based on a literal translation of the point names; however, they address the meaning of the point names in a superficial way only. Much is lost in translation and through lack of cultural understanding. In reality, the poetic nature of the point names embrace myriad subtleties and depths of meaning, which relate not only to the physical but also the emotional and spiritual aspects of their functions. Once qualified, a worthy practitioner will want to gain a fuller understanding of these aspects of the tradition. However, all of this is far beyond the remit of this book. Drawings and notations are geared towards remembering and recalling for the purpose of grasping the basics of the subject.

In the end, there is no single right way to learn. Instead I would encourage students to bring to this book the traditions of their chosen institute of learning, as well as their own individual hang ups, strengths and idiosyncrasies in learning.

The inspiration for this book came directly from my own need for a method by which to learn the point functions while in the second year of my acupuncture training. Daunted by the volume of 'bits' of information in front of me, and the knowledge that younger and brighter students than I were struggling with the task, I set out to find a way to learn just a single fact about each point on the Heart Channel. The result was a simple drawing, which proved so surprisingly easy to remember and recall that I continued adding more and more information until I had enough to pass the weekly test. This approach formed the basis for all subsequent drawings of the remaining channels.

Before too long fellow students were becoming intrigued and were requesting copies, especially in the lead up to exams. They proved to be very popular and I began to get approached by students from other classes, and even other colleges, who had seen or heard of the drawings at regional group meetings. Eventually I found myself taking bulk orders over the phone from people I didn't know.

The Chinese medical model in general, and the acupuncture point functions in particular, lend themselves to visual description. The Chinese written language is itself made up of pictograms that are, in essence, a highly stylised set of drawings. It could be said that at its heart, Chinese, more than probably any other language, encompasses the visual element within its form. The highly poetic and visual nature of the medical language make it a ready subject for translation into images.

I would like to think that this book of drawings, although inherently 'Western' in its approach, fits sympathetically with the traditions of Chinese medicine rather than imposing itself upon it.

I hear and I forget,
I see and I remember,
I do and I understand.

Confucius

The Acupuncture Points Functions Colouring Book is in no way a definitive guide to acupuncture point functions. It cannot and must not be used as a manual in itself for the treatment of patients. That can only be done safely within the context of a full diagnosis by a qualified practitioner.

How to use *The Acupuncture Points Functions Colouring Book*

Please take time to read these instructions, as they will enable you to get the most out of the book and help prevent you from making mistakes.

- The chapters are arranged, one per channel, in their traditional order according to the law of midday and midnight, but users can start with any channel to suit their curriculum or college.

- Start by reviewing the pathway of the channel to be learnt or revised, using the diagram at the start of each chapter, and then turn to the page of drawings so that the text and drawings can be viewed together.

- Read the 'Point functions' text for each point and then view the drawing that corresponds to it. Work through the text and drawings logically in sequence, from Entry to Exit Point, in order to help establish the points on each channel as a distinct group.

- The abbreviation CF stands for Causative/Constitutional Factor, which is a Five Element diagnostic term.

- Read the text relating to each point function and then colour in the drawings using colours that seem appropriate and have resonance for you. These will be different for each individual.

- Not every point on every channel is drawn. You can add in drawings of the points that are absent if they are required for your particular course.

- Embellish the drawings and add your own doodles and notes to flesh out the information at each point. Your own doodles, however basic, will make them significantly more memorable and real for you, and give your memory something to latch on to. You may also find it helpful to palpate the points as you go, to connect location with function.

- Use colour sparingly as too much indiscriminate colour can obscure rather than enhance the memory. It is often better to use colour to highlight specific key functions or associations, for example the colours associated with the Five Elements (red, yellow, green, blue, white) on point numbers to help recall which are element points. You may wish to substitute grey for white when marking Metal Element points as white will not be visible. You can also create your own colour codes – for example, Xi-Cleft Points could always be coloured purple.

- When using the drawings for revision, chose channels and points at random to be sure you can remember them out of sequence.

- Make a note of any points or functions you are consistently having trouble recalling. Go over these points and embellish them further with doodles or add more colours. Spending more time thinking about how to enhance them will help fix them in your memory.

- You may even find that there is a spacial aspect to your learning, for example points in the lower left quarter of a page are always harder for you to memorise and recall. These points should be significantly more 'overworked' than drawings in other sections of the page that you are finding easier to remember.

- If you are not a confident colourer, you may want to do a test run on a scan or photocopy before colouring into the book, to avoid mistakes.

Good luck, and happy colouring!

Key

A number of symbols recur throughout the drawings. The following are the most common. You can add and create your own.

Damp	Damp-Heat	Fire	Heat	Wind

Clear	Subdue	Strengthen	Tonify	

Entry/Exit Point	Junction Point	Mu Point	Sedation Point	Source Point

Heavenly	Spirit	Window of Heaven		

The Heart Channel

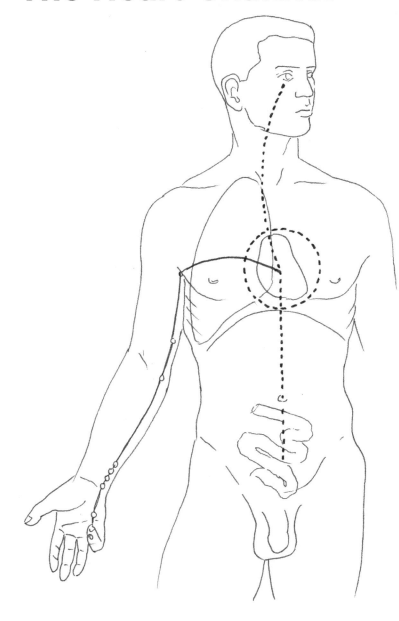

'The **Heart** holds the office of lord and sovereign.
The radiance of the Spirit stems from it.'

SU WEN CHAPTER 8

The **Fire Element** enables us to give and receive love with appropriate degrees of emotional closeness, to know how and when it is appropriate to open up or shut down to people, and to decide how much to open up to others in all different forms of relationships.

Physical areas particularly affected by Heart points

- Chest and upper *jiao*

- Anywhere on the Heart Channel

- Tongue (speech), throat and eye

- Connects with the Small Intestine (Organ and Channel/*Taiyang*), and can therefore influence the Bladder too

HEART POINT FUNCTIONS (HAND SHAOYIN)

He 1 Jiquan **Supreme Spring** *Entry Point*

Tonifying actions: Nourish Heart *Yin*. Strengthen and calm the Spirit. Activate the Channel.

Dispersing actions: Clear Empty Heat (and thus calm the Spirit). Expand and relax the chest. Remove obstructions from the Channel. Benefit the arm.

Main uses: Treat Fire (CF) and treat the Spirit. Entry Point (usually with Sp 21).

He 2 Qingling **Blue-Green Spirit**

Tonifying actions: Tonify Heart *Qi*. Strengthen the Spirit.

Dispersing actions: Expand and relax the chest. Regulate *Qi* and Blood (chest and Channel) and alleviate pain. Clear Heat (Channel). Calm the Spirit.

He 3 Shaohai **Lesser Sea** *Water Point, He Sea Point*

Tonifying actions: Strengthen and calm the Spirit. Activate the Channel.

Dispersing actions: Clear Heat from the Heart (and thus calm the Spirit). Remove obstructions from the Channel.

Main uses: Clear Heart Fire. Treat Fire (CF) and treat the Spirit.

He 4 Lingdao **Spirit Way** *Metal Point, Jing-River Point*

Tonifying actions: Strengthen the Spirit. Regulate the Heart/heart rhythm (and thus calm the Spirit). Benefit speech (sudden loss of voice).

Dispersing actions: Relax the muscles and sinews in the Channel.

Main uses: Treat Fire (CF) and treat the Spirit.

He 5 Tongli **Connecting Street** *Luo-Junction Point*

Tonifying actions: Tonify Heart *Qi*. Strengthen the Spirit. Benefit the tongue.

Dispersing actions: Clear Heart Fire and Empty Heat (and thus calm the Spirit). Benefit the Bladder.

Main uses: Treat Fire (CF), tonify Heart *Qi*, and treat the Spirit. As the Junction Point to strengthen the relationship with the Small Intestine (often with SI 7). Speech problems.

He 6 Yinxi **Yin Cleft** *Xi-Cleft Point*

Tonifying actions: Nourish Heart *Yin*. Strengthen and calm the Spirit. Alleviate sweating.

Dispersing actions: Clear Xu Heat in the Heart, Heat in the Blood and Heart Fire (and thus calm the Spirit). Regulate Heart *Qi* and Blood. Moderate acute conditions of Heart Organ and Channel.

Main uses: Nourish Heart *Yin*. Alleviate sweating (often with Kid 7). Treat acute conditions of Heart Organ and Channel.

He 7 Shenmen **Shen Gate** *Earth Point, Yuan-Source Point, Sedation Point, Shu-Stream Point*

Tonifying actions: Tonify Heart *Qi*. Nourish Heart Blood. Nourish Heart *Yin*. Strengthen and calm the Spirit.

Dispersing actions: Regulate Heart *Qi* and Blood. Open the orifices. Clear Heart Fire (and thus calm the Spirit).

Main uses: As Source Point to treat Fire (CF, often with SI 4). Treat the Spirit. For any Heart pattern, especially Xu patterns.

He 8 Shaofu **Lesser Treasury** *Fire Point, Horary Point, Ying-Spring Point*

Tonifying actions: Tonify Heart *Qi* and *Yang*, 'warm' the Heart and strengthen the Spirit.

Dispersing actions: Clear Heart Empty Heat, Heart (and Small Intestine) Fire, and Heart Phlegm-Fire (and thus calm the Spirit).

Main use: As Horary Point to treat Fire (CF, often with SI 5). Clear Heart Fire.

He 9 Shaochong **Lesser Surge** *Wood Point, Tonification Point, Jing-Well Point, Exit Point*

Tonifying actions: Tonify Heart *Qi* and *Yang*. Strengthen the Spirit.

Dispersing actions: Clear Heart Heat (and thus calm the Spirit). Relieve fullness in the Heart area. Open Heart orifices. Subdue internal Wind. Restore consciousness.

Main use: As Tonification Point to strengthen Fire (CF, usually with SI 3). Clear Heat.

Bl 15 Xinshu **Heart Back Shu Point**

Tonifying actions: Strengthen the Heart. Strengthen the Spirit. Stimulate the brain.

Dispersing actions: Clear Heart Heat. Regulate Heart *Qi* and Blood (and thus calm the Spirit).

Main uses: Treat Fire CF (usually with Bl 27). For any Heart pattern.

Bl 44 Shentang **Shen Hall**

Tonifying actions: Stabilise and strengthen the Spirit.

Dispersing actions: Regulate the Heart. Relax the chest. Clear Heat in the Heart (and thus calm the Spirit).

Main use: Treat Fire (CF) and treat the Spirit.

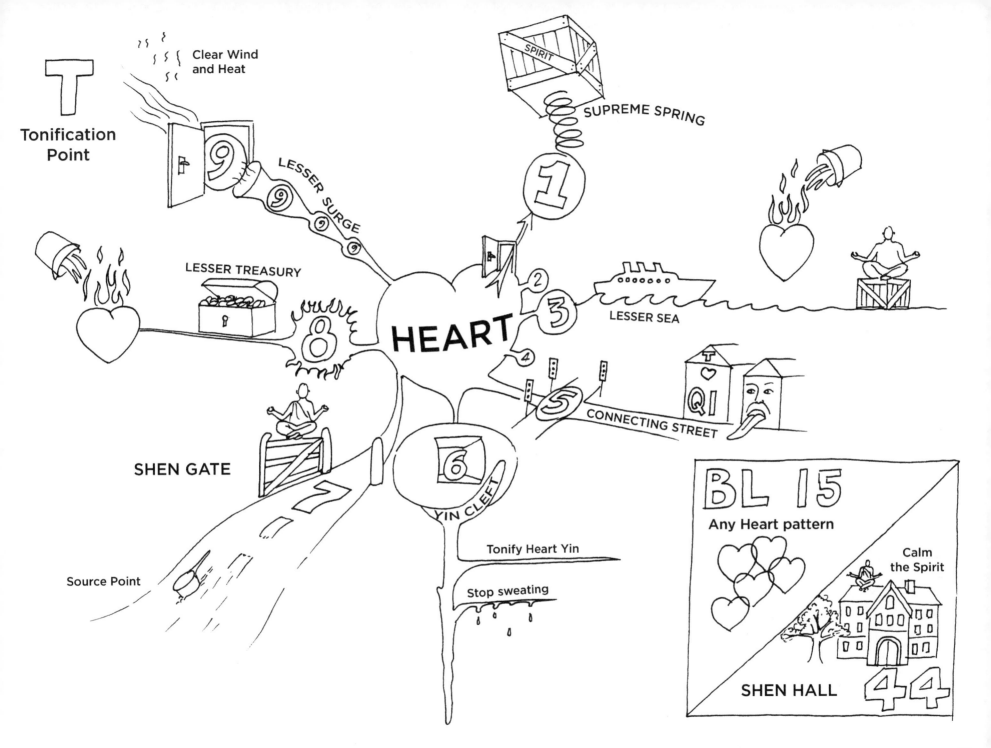

Tonification Point

Clear Wind and Heat

SPIRIT

SUPREME SPRING

LESSER SURGE

LESSER TREASURY

LESSER SEA

HEART

CONNECTING STREET

QI

SHEN GATE

YIN CLEFT

Tonify Heart Yin

Stop sweating

Source Point

BL 15

Any Heart pattern

Calm the Spirit

SHEN HALL

Notes

The Small Intestine Channel

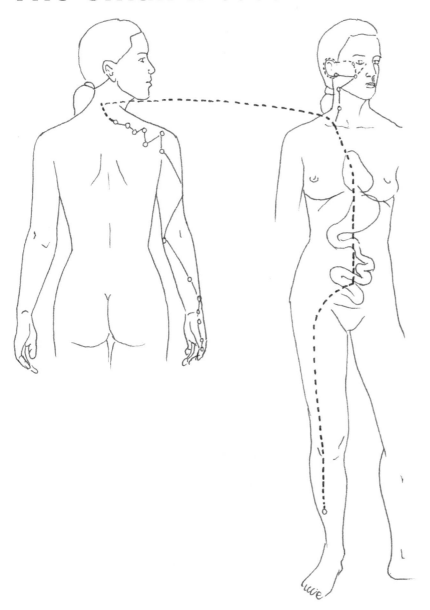

'The **Small Intestine** is responsible for receiving and making things thrive. Transformed Substances stem from it.'

SU WEN CHAPTER 8

The **Fire Element** enables us to give and receive love with appropriate degrees of emotional closeness, to know how and when it is appropriate to open up or shut down to people, and to decide how much to open up to others in all different forms of relationships.

Physical areas particularly affected by Small Intestine points

- Anywhere on the Small Intestine Channel

- Shoulder, neck, arm and wrist

- Connects with the Heart (Organ) and can therefore influence the chest

- Connects with the Stomach (Organ) and can therefore influence rebellious *Qi*

- Connects with the Bladder (Channel/Taiyang), and can therefore influence urination, the eyes and the spine and neck

- Connects with the Du Mai (Channel) and can therefore influence the spine and neck

- Connects with the Triple Burner and Gall Bladder (Channels), which strengthens its influence on the ears

SMALL INTESTINE POINT FUNCTIONS (HAND TAIYANG)

SI 1 Shaoze **Lesser Marsh** *Metal Point, Jing-Well Point, Entry Point*

Tonifying actions: Activate the Channel.

Dispersing actions: Expel Wind-Heat (fevers). Extinguish (internal) Wind and restore consciousness. Clear Heat (Channel) and benefit the sensory orifices. Remove obstructions from the Channel. Promote lactation and benefit the breasts.

Main uses: For breast abscess and swelling, and disorders of lactation (often with Ren 17). As the Entry Point.

SI 2 Qiangu **Front Valley** *Water Point, Ying-Spring Point*

Tonifying actions: Moisten the Small Intestine Organ or Channel. Benefit and moisten the ears, eyes and throat.

Dispersing actions: Clear Heat. Expel Wind-Heat (fevers). Remove obstructions from the Channel.

Main use: Clear Heat (Channel, Heart and Bladder).

SI 3 Houxi **Back Stream** *Wood Point, Tonification Point, Shu-Stream Point, Opening Point of Du Mai*

Tonifying actions: Tonify Small Intestine. Strengthen and clear the Spirit. Activate the Channel.

Dispersing actions: Regulate Du Mai and extinguish internal Wind. Expel external Wind. Remove obstructions from the Channel. Resolve Damp (used to treat Malaria).

Main use: As the Tonification Point to strengthen Fire (CF, usually with He 9). Treat the Spirit. As the Opening Point of Du Mai (often with Coupled Point Bl 62). Clear Wind from the spine and neck (acute stiff neck).

SI 4 Wangu **Wrist Bone** *Yuan-Source Point*

Tonifying actions: Tonify Small Intestine. Activate the Channel.

Dispersing actions: Remove obstructions from the Channel. Eliminate Damp-Heat (febrile diseases, jaundice).

Main uses: As the Source Point to strengthen Fire (CF, usually with He 7). Channel problems.

SI 5 Yanggu **Yang Valley** *Fire Point, Horary Point, Jing-River Point*

Tonifying actions: Tonify Small Intestine. Strengthen and clear the Spirit. Activate the Channel.

Dispersing actions: Clear Heat (and thus calm the Spirit). Eliminate Damp-Heat (swellings in neck). Remove obstructions from the Channel.

Main use: As the Horary Point to treat Fire (CF, usually with He 8). Treat the Spirit. Clear Heat (Heart Channel). Channel problems.

SI 6 Yanglao **Nourishing the Old** *Xi-Cleft Point*

Tonifying actions: Benefit the eyes (in deficiency conditions of Heart and Small Intestine).

Dispersing actions: Remove obstructions from the Channel. Relax tendons. (Name suggests a particular use for these problems if long-standing or associated with old age.)

SI 7 Zhizheng **Branch to the Heart Channel** *Luo-Junction Point*

Tonifying actions: Strengthen and calm the Spirit.

Dispersing actions: Expel Wind and Heat. Release the Exterior and stimulate sweating. Remove obstructions from the Channel.

Main uses: As the Junction Point to strengthen the relationship with Heart (often with He 5). Treat Fire (CF) by promoting the Small Intestine function of separating pure from impure. Treat the Spirit.

SI 8 Xiaohai **Small Sea** *Earth Point, Sedation Point, He Sea Point*

Dispersing actions: Remove obstructions from the Channel. Resolve Damp-Heat. Relax tendons.

Main use: As a local point for the elbow. (NB not considered very effective as He Sea Point to treat the Small Intestine Organ. Consider St 39, the Lower He Sea Point, instead.)

SI 9–10 and 13–15

Main use: Channel problems of the shoulder.

SI 9 Jianzhen **Upright Shoulder**

Tonifying actions: Activate the Channel. Benefit the shoulder.

Dispersing actions: Remove obstructions from the Channel. Benefit the shoulder.

SI 10 Naoshu **Upper Arm Shu Point**

Tonifying actions: Activate the Channel. Benefit the shoulder.

Dispersing actions: Remove obstructions from the Channel. Benefit the shoulder.

SI 11 Tianzong **Heavenly Ancestor**

Tonifying actions: Strengthen the Spirit. Activate the Channel. Benefit the shoulder.

Dispersing actions: Remove obstructions from the Channel. Benefit the Shoulder. Move *Qi* – opens the chest and lateral costal region. Facilitate lactation. Redirect rebellious *Qi* (cough).

Main use: Strengthen the Spirit (Fire CF).

SI 12 Bingfeng **Grasping the Wind**

Tonifying actions: Activate the Channel. Benefit the shoulder.

Dispersing actions: Remove obstructions from the Channel. Benefit the shoulder. Dispel Wind-Cold and Wind-Heat.

SI 13 Quyuan **Crooked Wall**

Tonifying actions: Activate the Channel. Benefit the shoulder.

Dispersing actions: Expel Wind (*Bi*). Remove obstructions from the Channel. Benefit the shoulder.

SI 14 Jianwaishu **Outside of the Shoulder Shu Point**

Tonifying actions: Activate the Channel. Benefit the shoulder.

Dispersing actions: Expel Wind (*Bi*). Remove obstructions from the Channel. Benefit the shoulder.

Continued on page 22

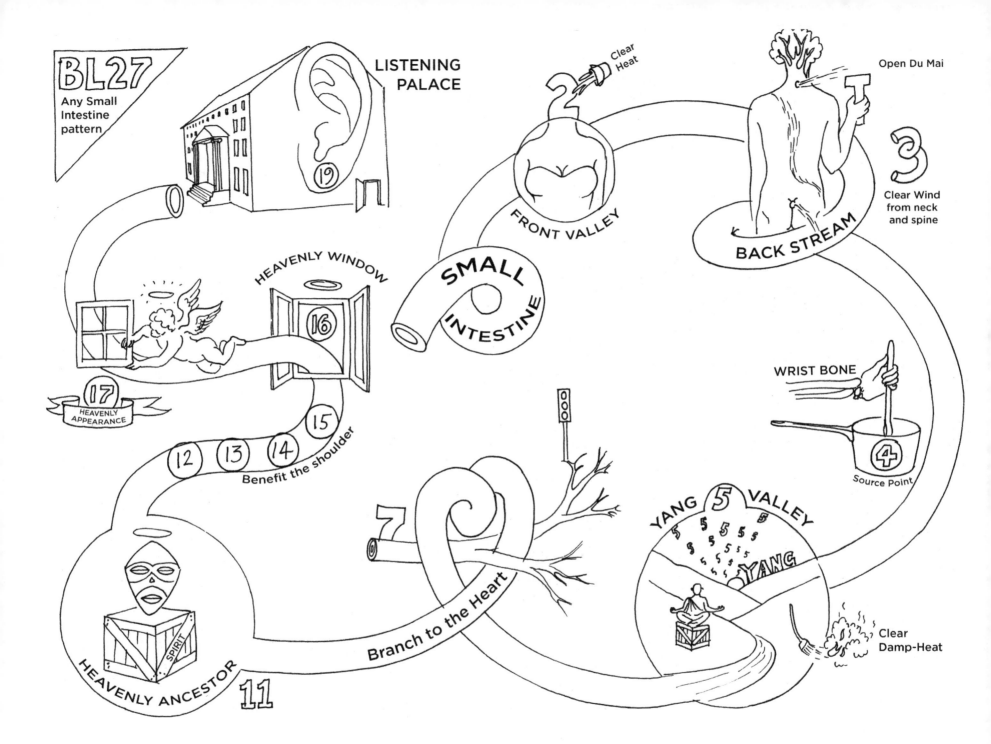

SI 15 Jianzhongshu Centre of the Shoulder Shu Point

Tonifying actions: Activate the Channel. Benefit the shoulder.

Dispersing actions: Remove obstructions from the Channel. Benefit the shoulder. Descend Lung *Qi*.

SI 16 Tianchuang Heavenly Window *Window of Heaven*

Tonifying actions: Unite *Qi* of Heaven and Earth.

Dispersing actions: Regulate the ascending and descending of *Qi* and calm the Spirit. Subdue Wind (internal). Benefit ears, throat and voice. Remove obstructions from the Channel.

Main use: As a Window of Heaven (Fire CF).

SI 17 Tianrong Heavenly Appearance *Window of Heaven*

Tonifying actions: Unite *Qi* of Heaven and Earth.

Dispersing actions: Subdue rebellious *Qi*. Resolve Damp and Heat and expel Fire-Poison. Benefit the ears, neck and throat.

Main use: As a Window of Heaven (Fire CF). Specific for severe acute tonsillitis.

SI 18 Quanliao Cheekbone Foramen

Dispersing actions: Expel Wind. Clear Heat. Relieve pain (local point).

SI 19 Tinggong Listening Palace *Exit Point*

Tonifying actions: Promote discerning and discriminating function of the Small Intestine. Strengthen and calm the Spirit. Benefit the ears.

Dispersing actions: Benefit the ear.

Main use: Exit Point (often with Bl 1). Strengthen and calm the Spirit (Fire CF). Benefit the ears (mainly in deficiency conditions).

Bl 27 Xiaochangshu Small Intestine Back Shu Point

Tonifying actions: Promote Small Intestine functions.

Dispersing actions: Resolve Damp. Clear Heat. Benefit urination. Regulate *Qi* of the Intestines and Bladder.

Main use: Treat Fire (CF, usually with Bl 15). Any Small Intestine pattern.

The Bladder Channel

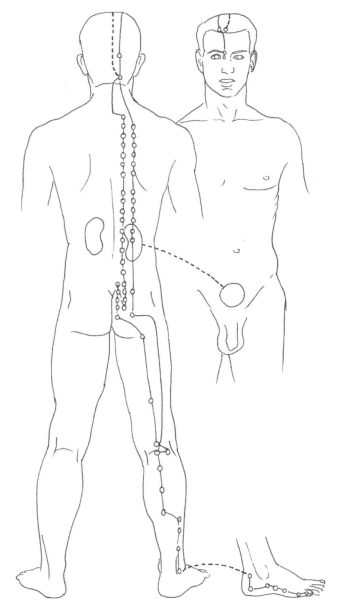

'The **Bladder** is responsible for the regions and cities. It stores the body fluids. The transformations of the *Qi* then give out their power.'

SU WEN CHAPTER 8

The **Water Element** enables us to notice danger and assess the extent of the risk it presents, reassure ourselves that we are safe, and take action to deal with risk.

Physical areas particularly affected by Bladder points

- Anywhere on the Bladder Channel, especially:

  - Spine from lumbar regions to shoulders and neck

  - Brain

  - Eyes, nose and head

  - Bladder, lower orifices and Uterus

- Connects with the Small Intestine, Triple Burner, Gall Bladder and Du Channels, which strengthens its effect on areas of the back and head

- Physical organs via the Back Shu Points

BLADDER POINT FUNCTIONS (FOOT TAIYANG)

Bl 1 Jingming Eyes Bright *Meeting Point of Bl, SI, and St, Entry Point, Point of the Yin and Yang Qiao Mai*

Tonifying actions: Tonify Bladder *Qi*. Strengthen the Spirit (Water CF). Brighten the eyes.

Dispersing actions: Expel Wind. Clear Heat. Brighten the eyes. Stop itching.

Main use: Entry Point (often with SI 19). Tonify Bladder *Qi* and strengthen the Spirit (Water CF). Eye diseases.

Bl 2 Zanzhu Collecting Bamboo

Tonifying actions: Brighten the eyes (e.g. when affected by symptoms of Liver deficiency).

Dispersing actions: Expel (external) Wind. Clear Heat. Subdue Liver *Yang*. Brighten the eyes. Alleviate pain. Clear the nose.

Main use: Eye problems. Clear the nose (often with LI 20 or *Yintang*).

Bl 7 Tongtian Penetrating Heavenly Connection

Dispersing actions: Subdue (internal) Wind. Subdue Liver *Yang*. Clear the nose.

Main use: Clear the nose. Vertex headaches.

Bl 10 Tianzhu Heavenly Pillar *Window of Heaven, Point of Sea of Qi*

Tonifying actions: Unite *Qi* of Heaven and Earth (Water CF). Strengthen the *Qi* of the Channel.

Dispersing actions: Expel (external) Wind. Subdue (internal) Wind. Subdue Liver *Yang*. Clear the Brain. Open the sense orifices. Remove obstructions from the Channel. Brighten the eyes. Regulate the low back.

Main use: Window of Heaven (Water CF). Channel problems (from deficiency or excess).

Bl 11 Dazhu Great Shuttle *Hui Point for Bones, Meeting Point of Bl and SI, Point to Release External Dragons, Point of Sea of Blood*

Tonifying actions: Nourish Blood. Firm the Exterior. Strengthen Bones.

Dispersing actions: Expel Wind and firm the Exterior. Remove obstructions from the Channel. Release External Dragons.

Main use: Nourish Blood. Strengthen Bones. Release External Dragons (with Du 20, Bl 23 and Bl 61).

Bl 12 Fengmen Wind Gate *Meeting Point of Bl and Du Mai*

Tonifying actions: Nourish Blood. Strengthen the *Wei Qi* and firm the Exterior.

Dispersing actions: Expel (external) Wind and release the Exterior. Descend and disseminate Lung *Qi*. Benefit the nose. Regulate the *Ying* and the *Wei Qi*.

Main use: Expel External Pathogenic Wind (often with cups).

Bl 13, Bl 14, Bl 15, Bl 18, Bl 19, Bl 20, Bl 21, Bl 22, Bl 23, Bl 25 Back Shu Points of Lung, Percardium, Heart, Liver, Gall Bladder, Spleen, Stomach, Triple Burner, Kidney and Large Intestine

Refer to point function information for relevant Organs. Bl 28 is given below.

Bl 16 Dushu Governor Back Shu Point *Back Shu Point for Du Mai*

Dispersing actions: Regulate the Heart. Move *Qi* and Blood. Regulate *Qi* in the chest and abdomen.

Bl 17 Geshu Diaphragm Back Shu Point *Hui Point for Blood*

Tonifying actions: Nourish Blood. Strengthen the Spirit.

Dispersing actions: Move Blood. Benefit the sinews (blood stagnation from long term *Bi* syndrome). Cool Blood. Stop bleeding. Calm the Spirit. Open the chest and diaphragm. Descend rebellious *Qi* (Stomach, diaphragm).

Main use: For all diseases of the Blood: nourish, cool or move Blood, and therefore calm and strengthen Spirit. Often used with Bl 18 and Bl 20, 'The Magnificent Six', to nourish Blood.

Bl 24 Qihaishu Sea of Qi Back Shu Point *(Note location behind Ren 6 Sea of Qi)*

Dispersing actions: Remove obstructions from the Channel. Regulate *Qi* and Blood in lower *jiao*, regulate menstruation.

Tonifying actions: Strengthen the lower back and legs.

Bl 26 Guanyuanshu Yuan Back Shu Point *(Note location behind Ren 4 Gate to the Yuan Qi)*

Tonifying actions: Strengthen the lower back.

Dispersing actions: Regulate *Qi* and Blood in lower *jiao*.

Bl 28 Pangguanshu Bladder Back Shu Point

Tonifying actions: Tonify Bladder *Qi*. Strengthen the lower back.

Dispersing actions: Regulate the Bladder. Resolve Damp and Damp-Heat in the lower *jiao*. Dispel stagnation in the lower *jiao* and the Channel. Open the Water Passages in the lower *jiao*.

Main uses: Strengthen Water CF (with Bl 23). Any Bladder pattern especially urinary problems. Low back pain.

Bl 30 Baihuanshu White Ring Transporting Point

Tonifying actions: Benefit the anus. Firm *Qi*. Strengthen lower back and legs.

Main use: Anal problems such as prolapse, haemorrhoids, faecal incontinence.

Bl 31 Shangliao Upper Foramen
Bl 32 Ciliao Second Foramen *(Has widest general actions of the four. Best of the points to tonify Kidneys and Jing)*
Bl 33 Zhongliao Central Foramen *(Most direct action on Bladder)*
Bl 34 Xialiao Lower Foramen *(Strongest action on genitals)*

Tonifying actions: Strengthen the lumbar region and knees. Warm the Kidneys. Nourish *Jing*.

Dispersing actions: Regulate lower *jiao* and facilitate urination and defecation. Regulate menstruation and resolve Damp (leucorrhoea) and Damp-Heat.

Continued on page 26

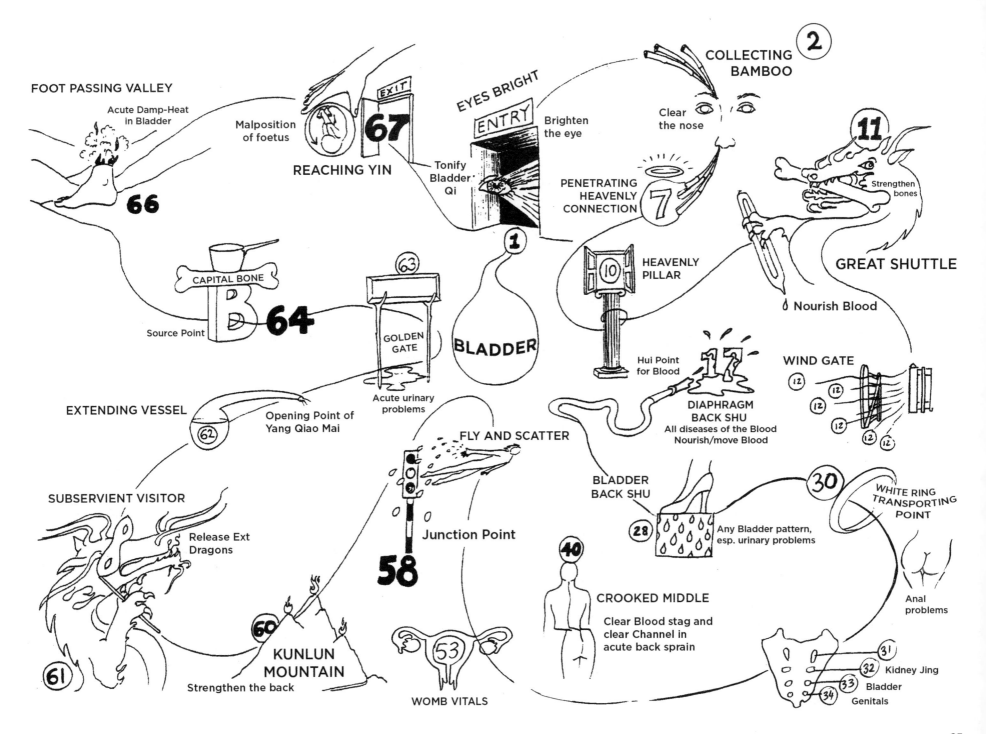

FOOT PASSING VALLEY

Acute Damp-Heat in Bladder

66

Malposition of foetus

REACHING YIN

EXIT

ENTRY

67

Tonify Bladder Qi

EYES BRIGHT

Brighten the eye

Clear the nose

COLLECTING BAMBOO ②

PENETRATING HEAVENLY CONNECTION 7

11

Strengthen bones

GREAT SHUTTLE

HEAVENLY PILLAR

10

Nourish Blood

CAPITAL BONE

B **64**

Source Point

63

GOLDEN GATE

Acute urinary problems

①

BLADDER

Hui Point for Blood

17

DIAPHRAGM BACK SHU

All diseases of the Blood Nourish/move Blood

WIND GATE

12 12 12 12 12 12

EXTENDING VESSEL

62

Opening Point of Yang Qiao Mai

FLY AND SCATTER

58

Junction Point

BLADDER BACK SHU

28

Any Bladder pattern, esp. urinary problems

30

WHITE RING TRANSPORTING POINT

SUBSERVIENT VISITOR

Release Ext Dragons

61

60

KUNLUN MOUNTAIN

Strengthen the back

40

CROOKED MIDDLE

Clear Blood stag and clear Channel in acute back sprain

Anal problems

53

WOMB VITALS

31

32 Kidney Jing

33 Bladder

34

Genitals

Bl 39 Weiyang **Crooked Yang**
Lower He Sea Point of TB

Tonifying actions: Stimulate the transformation and excretion of Fluids in the lower *jiao*. Benefit the Bladder.

Dispersing actions: Open the Water Passages in the lower *jiao*. Benefit the Bladder. Regulate the Triple Burner. Remove obstructions from the Channel.

Bl 40 Weizhong **Supporting Middle/ Crooked Middle** *Earth Point, He Sea Point*

Tonifying actions: Strengthen and stabilise Water (CF).

Dispersing actions: Clear Heat. Resolve Damp. Cool Blood. Clear Blood Stasis. Clear Summer Heat. Benefit the Bladder. Remove obstructions from the Channel.

Main uses: Acute back sprain (Bladder Channel). Skin diseases characterised by Heat and/or Damp.

Bl 42, Bl 43, Bl 44, Bl 47, Bl 48, Bl 49, Bl 50, Bl 51, Bl 52 **Outer Bladder Line Points of Lung, Pericardium, Heart, Liver, Gall Bladder, Spleen, Stomach, Triple Burner and Kidneys**

Refer to point function information for relevant organs.

Bl 53 Baohuang **Womb Vitals**

Tonifying actions: Strengthen the Bladder. Stimulate the transformation and excretion of fluids.

Dispersing actions: Open the Water Passages and regulate the lower *jiao*. Benefit urination. Remove obstructions from the Channel.

Bl 54 Zhibian **Lowermost Edge**

Tonifying actions: Strengthen Kidney *Qi*, low back and knees.

Dispersing actions: Remove obstructions from the Channel. Regulate urination. Treat haemorrhoids.

Main uses: Low back pain, sciatica, *Bi* syndrome affecting the legs (palpate for tenderness, along with Bl 53 and GB 30).

Bl 57 Chengshan **Supporting Mountain**

Dispersing actions: Relax tendons. Remove obstructions from the Channel. Move Blood. Clear Heat.

Main uses: Calf pain. Heel pain. Empirical point for treatment of haemorrhoids (as is Bl 58).

Bl 58 Feiyang **Fly and Scatter**
Luo-Junction Point

Tonifying actions: Strengthen the Kidneys.

Dispersing actions: Remove obstructions from the Channel. Subdue rebellious *Qi* from the head.

Main uses: Junction Point to strengthen the relationship with the Kidneys (often with Kid 4). Distal point for low back pain and for sciatica affecting Bladder and Gall Bladder Channels. Empirical point for treatment of haemorrhoids (as is Bl 57).

Bl 59 Fuyang **Instep** *Yang Xi-Cleft Point, Point of Yang Qiao Mai*

Tonifying actions: Invigorate *Yang Qiao Mai*.

Dispersing actions: Remove obstructions from the Channel.

Bl 60 Kunlun **Kunlun Mountain**
Fire Point, Jing-River Point

Tonifying actions: Strengthen the back.

Dispersing actions: Clear Heat and lower *Yang*. Subdue internal Wind. Remove obstructions from the Channel. Relax tendons. Move Blood. Promote labour.

Main use: Strengthen the back. Strengthen and warm Water CF (often with Kid 2). Distal point for obstructions (or rising *Yang*) affecting the Bladder Channel in low back, head, neck and shoulders.

Bl 61 Pucan **Subservient Visitor** *Point to Release External Dragons*

Main use: Release External Dragons (with Du 20, Bl 11 and Bl 23).

Bl 62 Shenmai **Extending Vessel**
Opening Point of Yang Qiao Mai

Tonifying actions: Strengthen Water (CF).

Dispersing actions: Subdue internal Wind and expel external Wind. Calm the Spirit. Benefit the eyes. Open *Yang Qiao Mai*. Remove obstructions from the Channel.

Main use: Opening Point of *Yang* Qiao Mai (with Coupled Point SI 3). Insomnia/somnolence (with Kid 6).

Bl 63 Jinmen **Golden Gate** *Xi-Cleft Point*

Tonifying actions: Strengthen the low back. Strengthen Water (CF).

Dispersing actions: Remove obstructions from the Channel. Subdue internal Wind.

Main use: Acute urinary problems characterised by Heat and pain.

Bl 64 Jinggu **Capital Bone** *Yuan-Source Point*

Tonifying actions: Tonify *Qi* of the Bladder and Kidneys and strengthen Water (CF). Strengthen the back. Strengthen the Spirit.

Dispersing actions: Subdue rebellious *Qi* and clear the head and eyes. Eliminate Wind (internal or external). Calm the Spirit.

Main use: As the Source Point to strengthen Water (CF, usually with Kid 3).

Bl 65 Shugu **Binding Bone** *Wood Point, Sedation Point, Shu-Stream Point*

Dispersing actions: Subdue rebellious *Qi* and clear the head and eyes. Clear Heat. Expel external Wind. Remove obstructions from the Channel (*Bi* syndrome).

Bl 66 Zutonggu **Foot Passing Valley** *Water Point, Horary Point, Ying-Spring Point*

Tonifying actions: Tonify *Qi* of the Bladder and strengthen Water (CF).

Dispersing actions: Clear Heat. Eliminate Wind. Clear the head (especially to dispel Damp). Calm the Spirit.

Main uses: Acute Damp-Heat in the Bladder (cystitis; e.g. with Kid 2 or Kid 10). As the Horary Point to treat Water (CF, usually with Kid 10).

Bl 67 Zhiyin **Reaching** *Yin Metal Point, Tonification Point, Jing-Well Point, Exit Point*

Tonifying actions: Tonify *Qi* of the Bladder and strengthen Water (CF).

Dispersing actions: Eliminate Wind (internal and external) and clear the head and eyes. Clear Heat. Turn the foetus. Facilitate labour.

Main use: As the Tonification Point to treat Water (CF, usually with Kid 7). To turn the foetus.

The Kidney Channel

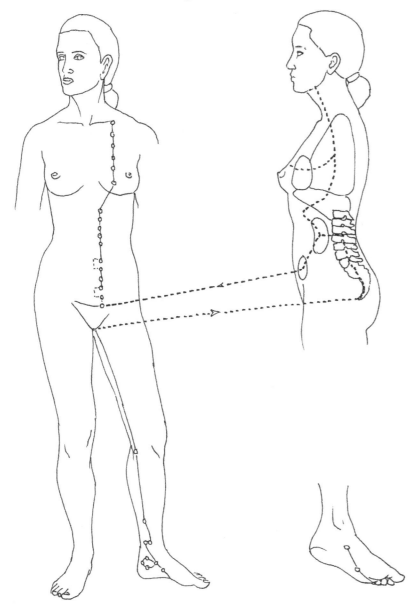

'The **Kidneys** are responsible for the creation of power. Skill and ability stem from them.'

SU WEN CHAPTER 8

The **Water Element** enables us to notice danger and assess the extent of the risk it presents, reassure ourselves that we are safe, and take action to deal with risk.

Physical areas particularly affected by Kidney points

Anywhere on the Kidney Channel, including:

- Knees

- Lower *jiao*, reproductive organs, bladder and kidneys

- Spine and brain

- Abdomen, chest and throat

- Ears

KIDNEY POINT FUNCTIONS
(FOOT SHAOYIN)

Kid 1 Yongquan **Bubbling Spring** *Wood Point, Sedation Point, Entry Point, Jing-Well Point*

Tonifying actions: Nourish *Yin*. Calm and strengthen the Spirit.

Dispersing actions: Clear Empty Heat. Subdue (internal) Wind. Descend excess *Yang*, Wind or Fire from the head. Calm the Spirit. Restore consciousness (windstroke).

Main uses: Clear Empty Heat due to *Yin* Xu. Descend Heat or Wind from the head. Calm the Spirit. Strengthen Water CF (maybe with Bl 1). Tonify the Kidneys.

Kid 2 Rangu **Blazing Valley** *Fire Point, Ying-Spring Point, Beginning Point of Yin Qiao Mai*

Tonifying actions: Warm and tonify Kidney *Yang*. Invigorate *Yang Qiao Mai*.

Dispersing actions: Clear Empty Heat. Cool Blood. Regulate the lower *jiao*.

Main uses: Clear Empty Heat. Cool Blood. Strengthen and warm Water CF (often with Bl 60).

Kid 3 Taixi **Greater Stream** *Shu-Stream Point, Yuan-Source Point, Earth Point*

Tonifying actions: Tonify Kidney *Yin, Yang, Jing* or *Yuan Qi*. Strengthen the lower back and knees.

Dispersing actions: Regulate the Uterus.

Main use: As the Source Point to strengthen Water (CF, usually with Bl 64). Tonify Kidney *Yin, Yang, Jing* or *Yuan Qi* (often with Ren 4 or Bl 23).

Kid 4 Dazhong **Great Cup** *Luo-Junction Point*

Tonifying actions: Strengthen the back. Calm and lift the Spirit. Strengthen the *Zhi* and dispel fear.

Main uses: As Junction Point to strengthen the relationship with the Bladder (often with Bl 58 or Bl 64). Chronic low back problems. Lift the Spirit (Water CF).

Kid 5 Shuiquan **Water Spring** *Xi-Cleft Point*

Tonifying actions: Tonify Kidneys.

Dispersing actions: Regulate *Qi* and Blood in *Ren* and *Chong Mai* and benefit menstruation. Benefit urination. Stop acute pain (urinary or menstrual).

Main uses: For acute and painful problems related to the Kidney Channel, e.g. acute cystitis, dysmenorrhoea.

Kid 6 Zhaohai **Shining Sea** *Opening Point of Yin Qiao Mai, Coupled Point of Ren Mai*

Tonifying actions: Nourish Kidney *Yin* and fluids. Strengthen and calm the Spirit. Invigorate *Yin Qiao Mai*. Benefit the eyes. Benefit the throat. Promote reception of *Qi* and open the chest. Promote the function of the Uterus.

Dispersing actions: Cool Blood. Regulate the Uterus and menstruation. Calm the Spirit.

Main uses: Nourish Kidney *Yin*. Open *Yin Qiao Mai* (often with Lu 7). With Lu 7 to open *Ren Mai*.

Kid 7 Fuliu **Returning Current** *Metal Point, Tonification Point, Jing-River Point*

Tonifying actions: Tonify the Kidneys (especially Kidney *Yang*). Strengthen the lower back. Open the Water Passages of the lower *jiao* and eliminate oedema. Regulate sweating from *Qi* or *Yin* deficiency (with He 6).

Dispersing actions: Promote sweating in attacks of EP Wind-Cold (with LI 4). Resolve Damp.

Main use: As the Tonification Point to treat Water CF (usually with Bl 67). Tonify Kidneys. Regulate sweating (with He 6). Promote sweating (with LI 4).

Kid 8 Jiaoxin **Intersection Reach** *Xi-Cleft Point of Yin Qiao Mai*

Dispersing actions: Regulate Blood in *Ren* and *Chong Mai*. Regulate menstruation. Remove obstructions from the Kidney and *Yin Qiao* Channels (abdominal masses in women). Stop (unilateral) abdominal pain.

Kid 9 Zhubin **Strengthening the River Bank** *Xi-Cleft Point of Yin Wei Mai*

Tonifying actions: Tonify Kidney *Yin*. Strengthen and calm the Spirit. Can be used at weeks 12, 24 and 36 of pregnancy to support Kidney *Qi* and foetal development.

Dispersing actions: Regulate *Yin Wei Mai* (links and stabilises Heart and Kidneys). Clear the Heart, open the chest and transform Phlegm. Calm the Spirit.

Main uses: Strengthen and calm the Spirit. In pregnancy to support foetal development.

Kid 10 Yingu **Yin Valley** *He Sea Point, Water Point, Horary Point*

Tonifying actions: Tonify Kidney *Yin*. Activate the Channel (local point).

Dispersing actions: Expel Damp from the lower *jiao*. Remove obstructions from the Channel (local point).

Main uses: Tonify Kidney *Yin*. Horary Point (often with Bl 66). Local point for Channel problems.

Kid 11–21

These are all points 'borrowed' by *Chong Mai*. Their actions reflect this.

Kid 12 Dahe **Great Brightness** *Meeting Point of Kidneys and Chong Mai*

Tonifying actions: Tonify Kidneys. Benefit and firm *Jing*.

Dispersing actions: Clear Heat (eyes – inner canthus).

Main use: Tonify and firm Kidney *Jing* (particularly in men).

Kid 13 Qixue **Qi Hole** *Meeting Point of Kidneys and Chong Mai*

Tonifying actions: Tonify Kidney *Qi* and *Jing*. Strengthen the Uterus. Consolidate *Chong* and *Ren Mai*.

Dispersing actions: Move *Qi* and Blood in lower *jiao*. Regulate *Chong Mai* and subdue 'running piglet *Qi*'. Clear Heat (eyes – inner canthus).

Main use: Tonify Kidney *Jing* (particularly in women).

Kid 14 Simian **Four Fullnesses** *Meeting Point of Kidneys and Chong Mai*

Tonifying actions: Nourish *Jing* and Marrow. Invigorate Blood in *Chong Mai*.

Dispersing actions: Move *Qi* and Blood in lower *jiao*. Regulate Uterus and menstruation. Regulate Water Passages and promote urination.

Main use: Move *Qi* and Blood in lower *jiao* and Uterus. (Name probably refers to the four accumulations of *Qi*, fluids, food and Blood.)

Continued on page 30

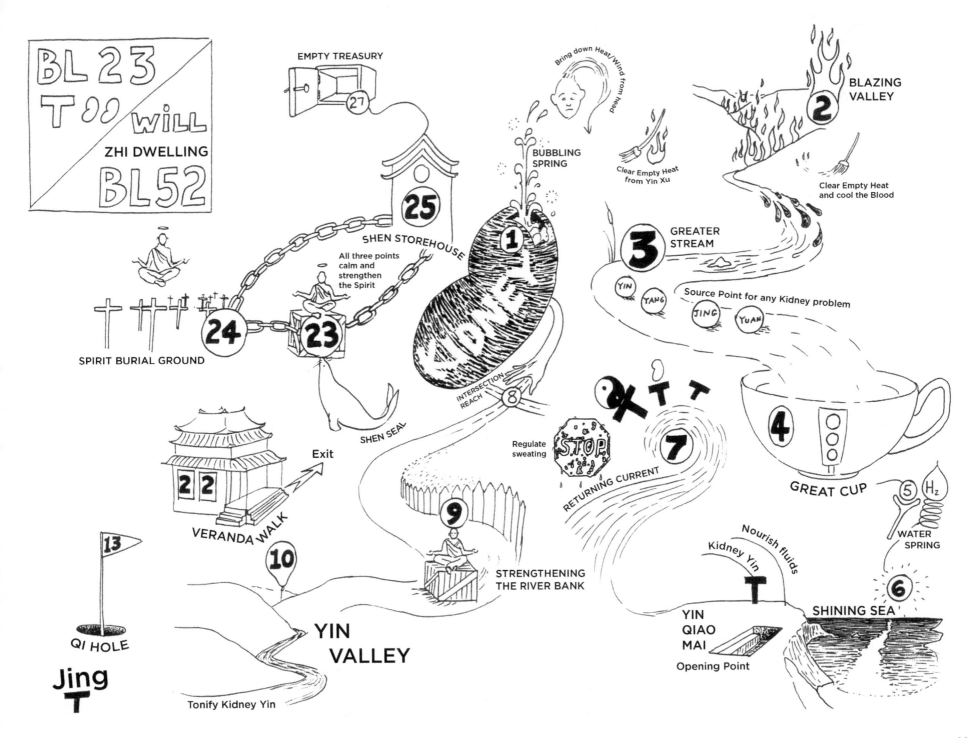

BL 23 T ∞ / will

ZHI DWELLING BL 52

EMPTY TREASURY

27

Bring down Heat/Wind from head

BLAZING VALLEY

2

Clear Empty Heat from Yin Xu

Clear Empty Heat and cool the Blood

BUBBLING SPRING

1

KIDNEY

SHEN STOREHOUSE

25

All three points calm and strengthen the Spirit

GREATER STREAM

3

YIN
YANG

Source Point for any Kidney problem

JING
YUAN

SPIRIT BURIAL GROUND

24   23

SHEN SEAL

INTERSECTION REACH

8

Regulate sweating

STOP

RETURNING CURRENT

7

4

GREAT CUP

5 H₂

WATER SPRING

VERANDA WALK

22

Exit

10

9

STRENGTHENING THE RIVER BANK

Nourish fluids

Kidney Yin

T

YIN QIAO MAI

Opening Point

6

WATER SPRING

SHINING SEA

13

QI HOLE

Jing
T

YIN VALLEY

Tonify Kidney Yin

29

Kid 16 Huangshu **Vitals Shu** *Meeting Point of Kidneys and Chong Mai*

Tonifying actions: Tonify the Kidneys. Benefit the Heart and calm the Spirit (Heart-Kidney axis).

Dispersing actions: Move *Qi* and Blood in lower *jiao*. Regulate (and warm) the Intestines.

Main use: Strengthen the Heart and Kidney Spirit.

Kid 20 Tonggu **Through the Valley** *Meeting Point of Kidneys and Chong Mai*

Tonifying actions: Harmonise the middle *jiao* (Kidney and Spleen functions).

Dispersing actions: Transform Phlegm in middle and upper *jiao*.

Kid 21 Youmen **Dark Gate** *Meeting Point of Kidneys and Chong Mai*

Tonifying actions: Fortify the Spleen. Harmonise the Stomach. Strengthen the Spirit (usually for Water CF).

Dispersing actions: Subdue rebellious *Qi* and stop vomiting (can be used for morning sickness). Spread the Liver *Qi*. Benefit the chest and breast.

Kid 22 Bulang **Veranda Walk** *Exit Point*

Tonifying actions: Strengthen/give confidence to the Spirit (any CF). Tonify the Kidneys.

Dispersing actions: Lower rebellious Lung and Stomach *Qi*.

Main use: Exit Point (usually with Pc 1 or Pc 2). Strengthen the Spirit.

Kid 23 Shenfeng **Shen Seal**

Tonifying actions: Strengthen/affirm the Spirit (any CF). Tonify the Kidneys.

Dispersing actions: Open the chest. Lower rebellious Lung and Stomach *Qi*. Benefit the breast

Main use: Strengthen and affirm the Spirit.

Kid 24 Lingxu **Spirit Burial Ground**

Tonifying actions: Strengthen/resurrect the Spirit. Tonify the Kidneys.

Dispersing actions: Open the chest. Lower rebellious Lung and Stomach *Qi*. Benefit the breast.

Main use: Strengthen and resurrect the Spirit.

Kid 25 Shencang **Shen Storehouse**

Tonifying actions: Strengthen/access the reserves of the Spirit. Tonify the Kidneys.

Dispersing actions: Open the chest and promote the descending of Lung *Qi*.

Main use: Strengthen and access the reserves of the Spirit. Local point for cough/wheezing/asthma from disharmony of Lung and Kidneys (e.g. with Lu 7 and Kid 6) or EP Wind (e.g. with LI 4 and Lu 7).

Kid 26 Yuzhong **Elegant Centre**

Tonifying actions: Tonify Kidneys and strengthen the Spirit.

Dispersing actions: Open the chest and lower rebellious Lung and Stomach *Qi*.

Kid 27 Shufu **Treasury Shu/Empty Treasury**

Tonifying actions: Strengthen/access the reserves of the Spirit. Tonify the Kidneys.

Dispersing actions: Promote the descending of Lung *Qi* and stop cough. Transform Phlegm. Harmonise Stomach *Qi* and stop vomiting (can be used for morning sickness).

Main use: Strengthen and access the reserves of the Spirit. Local point for asthma or bronchitis (e.g. with Lu 7 and Kid 6). Morning sickness (usually with Kid 6 and Kid 21).

Bl 23 Shenshu **Kidney Back Shu Point** *Point to Release External Dragons*

Tonifying actions: Tonify the Kidneys, fortify *Yang* and Nourish *Jing*. Firm Kidney *Qi*. Strengthen the lower back. Nourish Blood. Benefit Bones and Marrow. Benefit the ears and eyes.

Dispersing actions: Resolve Damp and Damp-Heat in the Bladder. Regulate the Water Passages and benefit urination.

Main use: Major point to tonify the Kidney. Release External Dragons (with Du 20, Bl 11 and Bl 61).

Bl 52 Zhishi **Zhi Dwelling**

Tonifying actions: Tonify the Kidneys and *Jing*. Strengthen the back. Strengthen the Will (*Zhi*).

Dispersing actions: Regulate urination.

Main use: Reinforce the Will (*Zhi*).

The Pericardium Channel

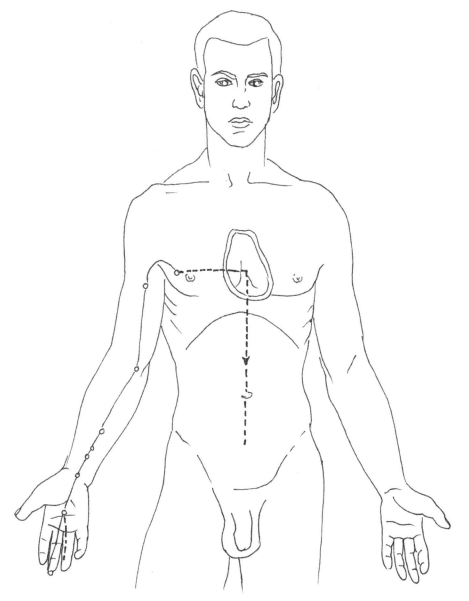

'The **Pericardium** represents the civil servants. From them come joy and pleasure.'

SU WEN CHAPTER 8

The **Fire Element** enables us to give and receive love with appropriate degrees of emotional closeness, to know how and when it is appropriate to open up or shut down to people, and to decide how much to open up to others in all different forms of relationships.

Physical areas particularly affected by Pericardium points

- Chest and upper *jiao*

- Heart

- Stomach

- Anywhere on the Pericardium Channel

PERICARDIUM POINT FUNCTIONS (HAND JUEYIN)

Pc 1 Tianchi Heavenly Pond *Window of Heaven, Entry Point, Meeting Point of Pc and Liver, TB and GB*

Tonifying actions: Unite the *Qi* of Heaven and Earth. Strengthen the Spirit/*Shen* and Heart Protector.

Dispersing actions: Open the chest, transform Phlegm and descend rebellious *Qi*. Regulate *Qi*. Dissipate nodules. Benefit the breasts (Heat, stagnation) and facilitate lactation (NB rarely possible to needle on a woman).

Main use: Window of Heaven (Fire CF; often with TB 16). Entry Point (usually with Kid 22).

Pc 2 Tianquan Heavenly Spring

Tonifying actions: Nourish the Heart and Heart Protector. Strengthen and calm the Spirit.

Dispersing actions: Open the chest. Move Blood and *Qi*. Alleviate pain (chest, upper back, shoulder, shoulder blade).

Main use: Nourish the Heart and Heart Protector. Strengthen and calm the Spirit. (May be used as an alternative to Pc 1 as Window of Heaven on women.)

Pc 3 Quze Crooked Marsh *Water Point, He Sea Point*

Tonifying actions: Strengthen and calm the Spirit.

Dispersing actions: Clear Heat (from the Heart) and Summer Heat. Cool Blood. Expel Fire-Poison. Move *Qi* and Blood in the chest. Calm the Spirit. Harmonise the Stomach and Intestines and stop vomiting. Remove obstructions from the Channel.

Main use: Clear Heat from the Heart.

Pc 4 Ximen Cleft Gate *Xi-Cleft Point*

Tonifying actions: Strengthen and calm the Spirit.

Dispersing actions: Invigorate/move Blood and dispel stasis. Stop pain. Cool Blood. Calm and regulate the Heart. Calm the Spirit. Remove obstructions from the Channel.

Main use: Regulate Blood for acute pain from Heart Blood stagnation.

Pc 5 Jianshi Intermediary *Metal Point, Jing-River Point, Meeting of Three Yin Channels of the Arm*

Tonifying actions: Strengthen the *Qi* of the chest: Heart, Heart Protector and Lung (rarely used as a Metal Point).

Dispersing actions: Resolve Phlegm in the Heart. Open the chest. Calm the Spirit. Harmonise the Stomach and subdue rebellious *Qi*. Invigorate Blood and regulate menstruation.

Main use: Resolve Phlegm in the Heart (often with St 40).

Pc 6 Neiguan Inner Gate *Luo-Junction Point, Opening Point of Yin Wei Mai, Coupled Point of Chong Mai*

Tonifying actions: Strengthen Heart Protector and upper *jiao*. Strengthen the relationship with the Triple Burner. Strengthen the Spirit.

Dispersing actions: Open the chest. Regulate Heart *Qi* and Blood. Calm the Spirit. Move Liver *Qi*. Harmonise the Stomach.

Main uses: Open the chest. Harmonise the Stomach. Strengthen and calm the Spirit. Junction Point to strengthen relationship with Heart Protector (often with TB 5). Opening Point of *Yin Wei Mai* (often with Coupled Point Sp 4).

Pc 7 Daling Great Burial Mound *Earth Point, Yuan-Source Point, Sedation Point, Shu-Stream Point*

Tonifying actions: Strengthen the Heart Protector and Heart. Strengthen the Spirit.

Dispersing actions: Clear Heat and toxic Heat. Calm the Spirit. Harmonise the Stomach and Intestines. Remove obstructions from the Channel (local).

Main use: As Source Point to strengthen Fire CF (usually with TB 4). Strengthen and calm the Spirit.

Pc 8 Laogong Palace of Weariness *Fire Point, Horary Point, Ying-Spring Point, Exit Point*

Tonifying actions: Strengthen/warm/enliven the Heart Protector. Strengthen the Spirit.

Dispersing actions: Clear Heart Fire. Calm the Spirit. Remove obstructions from the Channel (local).

Main uses: Horary Point to strengthen Fire CF (usually with TB 6). Clear Heart Fire.

Pc 9 Zhongchong Central Surge *Wood Point, Tonification Point, Jing-Well Point*

Tonifying actions: Strengthen the Heart Protector. Strengthen the Spirit.

Dispersing actions: Clear Heat. Expel Wind. Restore consciousness. Calm the Spirit.

Main use: Tonification point to strengthen Fire CF (usually with TB 3).

Bl 14 Jueyinshu Pericardium Back Shu Point

Tonifying actions: Strengthen the Heart Protector and Heart. Strengthen the Spirit.

Dispersing actions: Regulate the Heart. Open the chest.

Main uses: Back Shu Point to treat Fire CF (often with Bl 22). Tonify the Heart Protector and Heart. Regulate the Heart.

Bl 43 Gaohuangshu Vitals Back Shu Point

Tonifying actions: Strengthen *Yuan Qi*. Nourish *Jing*. Strengthen deficiency. Strengthen the Spirit. Nourish Lung *Yin*, calm (deficiency) asthma and cough.

Dispersing actions: Resolve Phlegm (in the Heart) and calm the Spirit.

Main use: Strengthen Fire CF. Strengthen deficiency (especially in/after chronic illness).

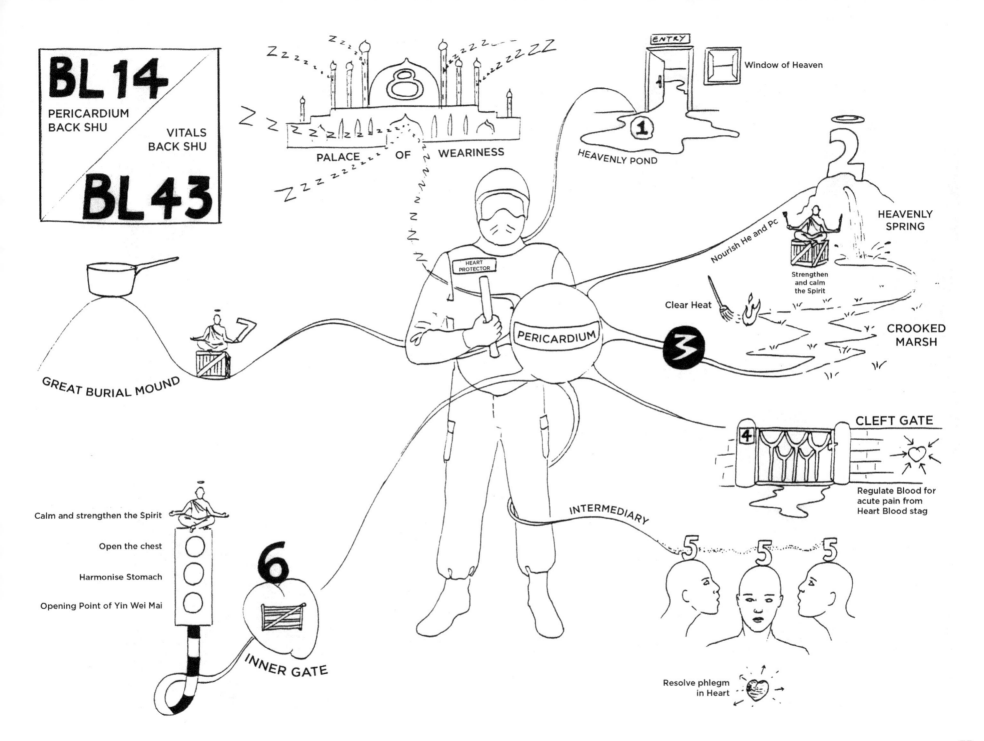

BL 14
PERICARDIUM BACK SHU

VITALS BACK SHU

BL 43

PALACE OF WEARINESS

Window of Heaven

HEAVENLY POND

HEAVENLY SPRING

Nourish He and Pc

Strengthen and calm the Spirit

Clear Heat

CROOKED MARSH

PERICARDIUM

HEART PROTECTOR

GREAT BURIAL MOUND

CLEFT GATE

Regulate Blood for acute pain from Heart Blood stag

INTERMEDIARY

Calm and strengthen the Spirit

Open the chest

Harmonise Stomach

Opening Point of Yin Wei Mai

INNER GATE

Resolve phlegm in Heart

Notes

The Triple Burner Channel

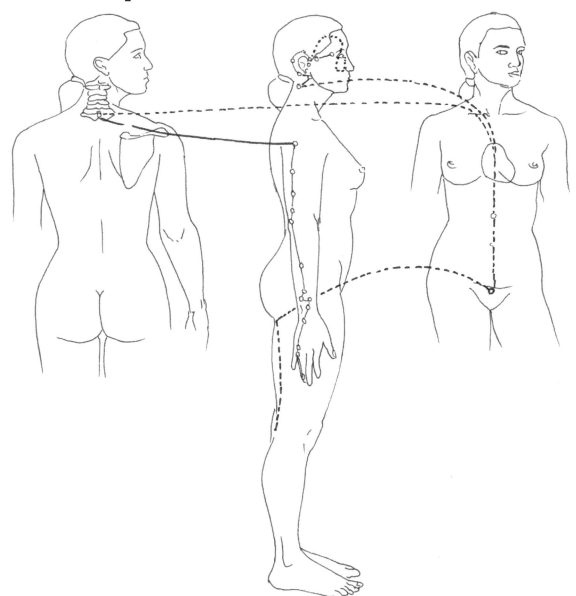

'The **Triple Burner** is responsible for the opening up of passages and irrigation. The regulation of fluids stems from it.'

SU WEN CHAPTER 8

The **Fire Element** enables us to give and receive love with appropriate degrees of emotional closeness, to know how and when it is appropriate to open up or shut down to people, and to decide how much to open up to others in all different forms of relationships.

Physical areas particularly affected by Triple Burner points

- Anywhere on the Triple Burner Channel

- Head, eye, ear and jaw

- Shoulder, neck, arm and wrist

- Connects with the Small Intestine and Gall Bladder Channels, which strengthens its influence on the shoulder, ears and head

- Connects with the Large Intestine Channel, which strengthens its influence on the shoulder

TRIPLE BURNER POINT FUNCTIONS (HAND SHAOYANG)

TB 1 Guanchong **Surging Pass** *Metal Point, Jing-Well Point, Entry Point*

Tonifying actions: Activate the Channel.

Dispersing actions: Clear Heat (in the Pericardium and in febrile diseases). Expel (external) Wind. Expel Wind-Heat. Benefit the ears and tongue. Remove obstructions from the Channel.

TB 2 Yemen **Fluids Gate** *Water Point, Ying-Spring Point*

Tonifying actions: Generate fluids. Moisten dryness. Moisten the throat.

Dispersing actions: Clear Heat and Wind-Heat (head and upper *jiao*, in febrile diseases). Regulate *Shaoyang*. Benefit the ears. Remove obstructions from the Channel.

TB 3 Zhongzhu **Middle Islet** *Wood Point, Tonification Point, Shu-Stream Point*

Tonifying actions: Strengthen the Triple Burner. Lift the Spirit.

Dispersing actions: Clear Heat and Wind-Heat (head and eyes in febrile diseases). Regulate *Shaoyang*. Subdue Liver *Yang*. Move Liver *Qi*. Benefit the ears. Remove obstructions from the Channel.

Main use: Tonification point to strengthen Fire CF (usually with Pc 9). Eye and ear problems from Liver *Yang* Rising or EP Wind-Heat.

TB 4 Yangchi **Yang Pond** *Yuan-Source Point*

Tonifying actions: Strengthen the Triple Burner. Promote fluid transformation. Benefit *Yuan Qi*. Strengthen *Yang*. Tonify *Chong* and *Ren Mai*.

Dispersing actions: Relax tendons. Clear Heat (Channel and febrile diseases). Regulate *Shaoyang*. Benefit the ears. Remove obstructions from the Channel.

Main use: As the Source Point to strengthen Fire CF (usually with Pc 7).

TB 5 Waiguan **Outer Gate** *Luo-Junction Point, Opening Point of Yang Wei Mai, Coupled Point of Dai Mai*

Tonifying actions: Strengthen the Triple Burner and the relationship with the Heart Protector. Strengthen the Spirit.

Dispersing actions: Expel Wind-Heat. Release the Exterior. Subdue Liver *Yang*. Benefit the head and ears. Regulate *Shaoyang*. Remove obstructions from the Channel.

Main use: Junction Point to strengthen the relationship with the Heart Protector (often with Pc 6). Release the Exterior and clear Wind-Heat (often with LI 4). Ear problems from Liver *Yang* Rising or EP Wind-Heat (often with TB 17). Opening Point of *Yang Wei Mai* to regulate *Shaoyang* (with Coupled Point GB 41).

TB 6 Zhigou **Branching Ditch** *Fire Point, Horary Point, Jing-River Point*

Tonifying actions: Strengthen the Triple Burner.

Dispersing actions: Regulate *Qi* and Clear Heat in the three *jiao*. Move the stool. Expedite lactation. Expel Wind. Remove obstructions from the Channel (with GB 34 affects flanks; with GB 31 clears Wind/Heat/Damp in skin complaints).

Main use: Horary Point to treat Fire CF (usually with Pc 8). Clear Wind and Heat.

TB 7 Huizong **Assembly of the Ancestors** *Xi-Cleft Point*

Tonifying actions: Strengthen the Triple Burner.

Dispersing actions: Remove obstructions from the Channel. Benefit the ears. Stop pain.

TB 8 Sanyangluo **Three** *Yang* **Connecting** *Meeting Point of Three Yang Channels of Arm*

Tonifying actions: Activate the Channel(s).

Dispersing actions: Remove obstructions from the Channel(s). Benefit the throat and ears.

TB 10 Tianjing **Heavenly Well** *Earth Point, Sedation Point, He Sea Point*

Tonifying actions: Strengthen the Triple Burner. Activate the Channel. Strengthen the Spirit.

Dispersing actions: Resolve Damp and Phlegm and dissipate nodules (Channel and chest). Remove obstructions and clear Heat from the Channel. Subdue rebellious (Liver/Gall Bladder) *Qi*. Calm the Spirit.

TB 13 Naohui **Upper Arm Convergence**

Tonifying actions: Activate the Channel.

Dispersing actions: Remove obstructions from the Channel.

TB 14 Jianliao **Shoulder Foramen**

Tonifying actions: Activate the Channel. Benefit the shoulder.

Dispersing actions: Remove obstructions from the Channel. Benefit the shoulder.

TB 15 Tianliao **Heavenly Foramen**

Tonifying actions: Activate the Channel. Benefit the shoulder.

Dispersing actions: Remove obstructions from the Channel. Benefit the shoulder. Open the chest and regulate *Qi*.

Main use of TB 14–15: Benefit the shoulder.

TB 16 Tianyou **Heavenly Window** *Window of Heaven*

Tonifying actions: Strengthen the Triple Burner and unite *Qi* of Heaven and Earth.

Dispersing actions: Regulate the ascending and descending of *Qi*, subdue rebellious *Qi* and Liver *Yang*.

Main use: Window of Heaven to treat Fire CF (often with Pc 1 or Pc 2).

TB 17 Yifeng **Wind Screen** *Meeting Point of TB and GB*

Tonifying actions: (Activate the Channel – rarely tonified.)

Dispersing actions: Expel Wind. Clear Heat. Benefit the ears and face. Remove obstructions from the Channel.

Main use: Benefit the ears.

TB 21 Ermen **Ear Gate**

Dispersing actions: Expel Wind. Clear Heat. Benefit the ears.

Continued on page 38

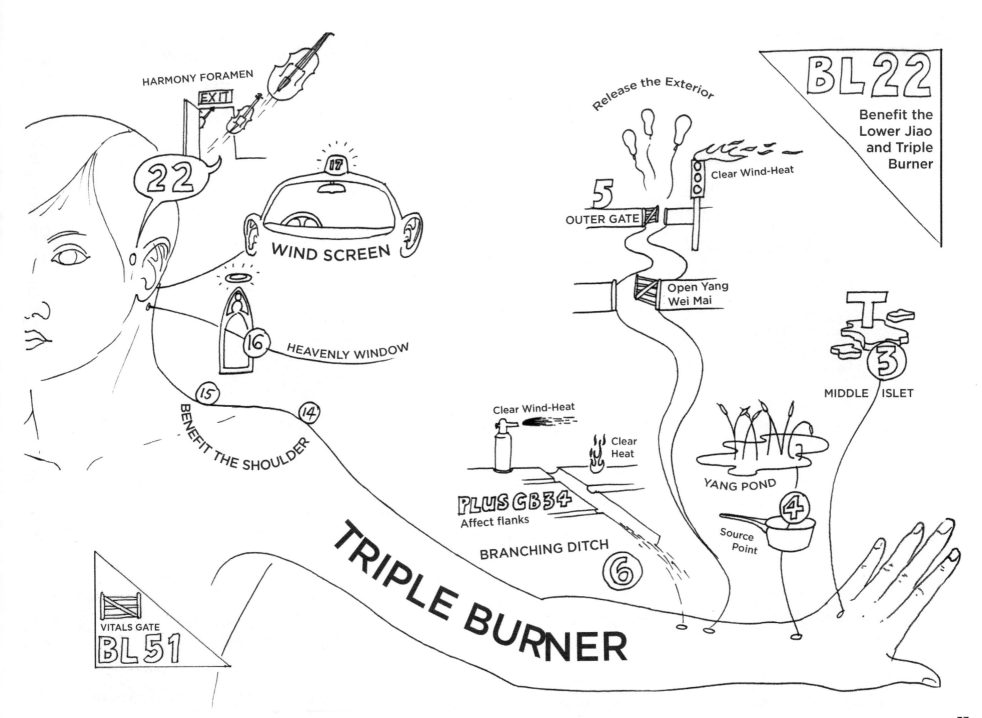

TB 22 Heliao **Harmony Foramen** *Exit Point*

Tonifying actions: (Rarely tonified except as Exit Point, according to pulse.)

Dispersing actions: Expel Wind (local).

Main use: Exit Point (often with GB 1).

TB 23 Sizhukong **Silk Bamboo Hollow**

Dispersing actions: Expel Wind. Brighten the eyes. Stop pain.

Bl 22 Sanjiaoshu **Triple Burner Back Shu Point**

Tonifying actions: Strengthen the Triple Burner and stimulate the transformation of fluids in the lower *jiao*.

Dispersing actions: Resolve Damp in the lower *jiao*. Open the Water Passages. Regulate the transformation of fluids in the lower *jiao*.

Main use: As the Back Shu point to treat Fire (CF). Strengthen/regulate metabolism of fluids.

Bl 51 Huangmen **Vitals Gate**

Tonifying actions: Strengthen the Triple Burner and the lower *jiao*.

Dispersing actions: Regulate the Triple Burner. Ensure the smooth spread of Triple Burner *Qi* to the Heart region. Dispel stagnation and benefit the breasts.

Main use: Outer Back Shu point used to strengthen the Spirit (Pericardium and Triple Burner Fire CFs), often with Bl 14 or Bl 43.

The Gall Bladder Channel

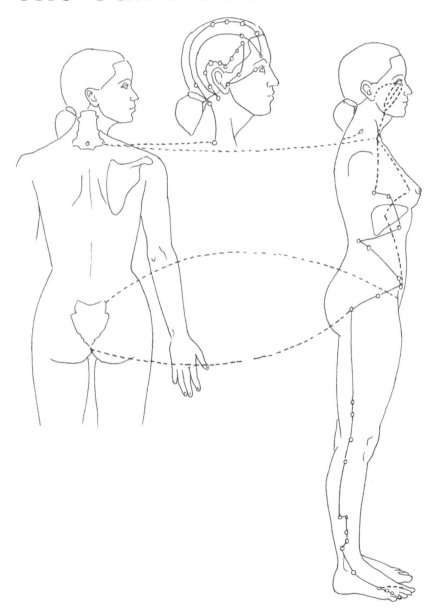

'The **Gall Bladder** is responsible for what is just and exact. Determination and decision stem from it.'

SU WEN CHAPTER 8

The **Wood Element** enables us to appropriately assert ourselves in the world, to have a clear vision of our own unique path in life, to have structures and boundaries in order that the path can unfold and make plans and decisions.

Physical areas particularly affected by Gall Bladder points

- Anywhere on the Gall Bladder Channel, especially:

  ◦ Head, eyes and ears

  ◦ Shoulders

  ◦ Flanks and waist

  ◦ Hips

  ◦ Lateral side of legs

  ◦ Liver and Gall Bladder

- Stomach and Heart

GALL BLADDER POINT FUNCTIONS (FOOT SHAOYANG)

GB 1 Tongziliao **Pupil Foramen** *Entry Point, Meeting Point of SI, GB and TB*

Tonifying actions: Brighten the eyes.

Dispersing actions: Expel external Wind. Clear Heat. Clear (Liver) Fire and Rising *Yang*. Brighten the eyes.

Main use: Entry Point. Local point for eye problems and temporal headaches.

GB 2 Tinghui **Hearing Assembly**

Dispersing actions: Remove obstructions from the Channel. Expel external Wind. Clear Heat. Benefit the ears.

GB 4–GB 12

The Channels GB, TB, Bl, St, and LI meet in various combinations at these points.

Main uses: Migraine, ear problems, facial and jaw problems, neck pain, etc. caused by Liver *Yang* Rising, Liver Fire or Liver Wind.

GB 8 Shuaigu **Leading Valley** *Meeting Point of GB and Bl*

Dispersing actions: Subdue Liver *Yang*. Eliminate Wind (internal and external). Benefit the ears. Remove obstructions from the Channel. Harmonise the Stomach and subdue rebellious Stomach *Qi*.

GB 9 Tianchong **Heavenly Surge** *Meeting Point of GB and Bl*

There are some textual indications that this point should be a Window of Heaven.

Tonifying actions: Strengthen the Spirit.

Dispersing actions: Subdue Liver *Yang*. Subdue internal Wind. Calm spasms. Resolve Damp and Phlegm and clear Heat in the head. Calm the Spirit.

Main use: Strengthen and/or calm the Spirit.

GB 12 Wangu **Completed Bone** *Meeting Point of GB and Bl*

Dispersing actions: Subdue Liver *Yang*. Eliminate Wind (internal and external). Calm the Spirit.

Main uses: Local point for headaches. Often used for insomnia from Liver *Yang* Rising or Liver Fire (with Bl 18 and Bl 19).

GB 13 Benshen **Shen Source** *Point of Yang Wei Mai*

Tonifying actions: Strengthen the Spirit. Gather *Jing* to the head (maybe with Ren 4).

Dispersing actions: Calm the Spirit. Subdue Liver *Yang*. Subdue internal Wind. Resolve Phlegm. Clear the brain.

Main uses: For mental and emotional disturbance and in psychiatric practice. Calm the Spirit (often with Du 24). Strengthen the Spirit. Stabilise the emotions.

GB 14 Yangbai **Yang White** *Meeting Point of GB, TB, St, and LI, Point of Yang Wei Mai*

Dispersing actions: Subdue Liver *Yang*. Eliminate Wind (internal and external). Brighten the eyes.

Main use: Local point for frontal headaches, facial paralysis and eye pain.

GB 15 Toulinqi **Head Overlooking Tears** *Meeting Point of GB and Bl, Point of Yang Wei Mai*

Tonifying actions: Strengthen the Spirit. Balance the emotions.

Dispersing actions: Calm the Spirit. Balance the emotions. Subdue Liver *Yang*. Subdue internal Wind. Brighten the eyes.

Main uses: For mood swings. Calm and/or strengthen and calm the Spirit.

GB 16 Muchuang **Eye Window** *Point of Yang Wei Mai*

Tonifying actions: Strengthen the Spirit.

Dispersing actions: Expel external Wind. Brighten the eyes. Calm the Spirit.

GB 18 Chengling **Receiving Spirit** *Point of Yang Wei Mai*

Tonifying actions: Strengthen the Spirit.

Dispersing actions: Calm the Spirit. Subdue Liver *Yang*. Benefit the nose. Descend Lung *Qi*.

Main use: Calm and/or strengthen and calm the Spirit (the *Ling*). (Can be used for obsessional thoughts and dementia.)

GB 20 Fengchi **Wind Pond** *Meeting Point of GB and TB, Meeting Point of Yang Wei Mai and Yang Qiao Mai*

Tonifying actions: Nourish Marrow and clear the brain.

Dispersing actions: Eliminate Wind (internal and external). Subdue Liver *Yang*. Clear Heat. Brighten the eyes. Benefit the ears. Remove obstructions from the Channel.

Main use: Head, neck or eye problems arising from Liver *Yang* Rising, external or internal Wind.

GB 21 Jianjing **Shoulder Well** *Meeting Point of GB and TB, Point of Yang Wei Mai*

Tonifying actions: Stimulate the descending of *Qi* and promote delivery and lactation. Stimulate the descending of Lung *Qi*.

Dispersing actions: Relax tendons. Regulate the Liver *Qi* and subdue Liver *Yang*. Resolve Phlegm and dissipate nodules. Remove obstructions from the Channel. Benefit the breasts and promote lactation.

Main uses: Neck, chest and shoulder problems from Liver pathologies. Promote delivery and lactation.

GB 24 Riyue **Sun and Moon** *Front Mu Point of GB*

Tonifying actions: Strengthen the Spirit.

Dispersing actions: Resolve Damp-Heat. Smooth *Qi* of Liver and Gall Bladder. Subdue rebellious *Qi* and harmonise the middle *jiao*. Calm the Spirit.

Main uses: To clear Liver *Qi* Stagnation. To resolve Damp-Heat (often with GB 34 and LI 11).

GB 25 Jingmen **Capital Gate** *Front Mu Point of Kid*

Tonifying actions: Tonify the Kidneys. Strengthen the lower back. Fortify the Spleen and regulate the Intestines.

Dispersing actions: Regulate the Water Passages of the lower *jiao*.

Main uses: To assist the mutual relationship between the Kidneys and Spleen (problems of digestion and of water metabolism). Renal colic. Hip pain.

Continued on page 42

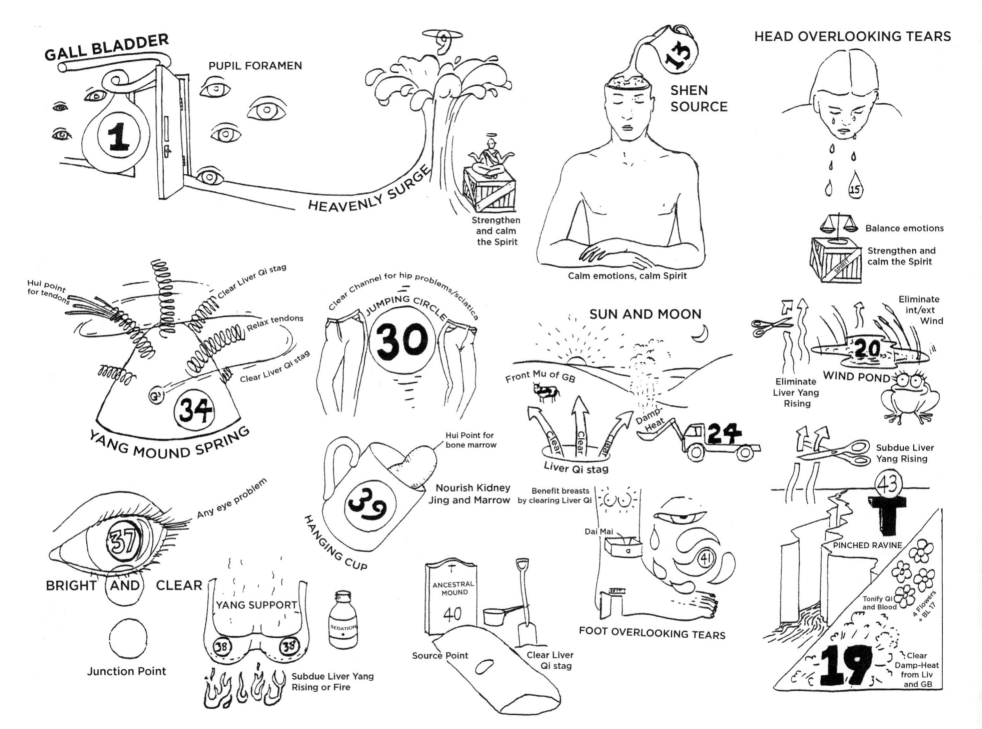

GALL BLADDER

PUPIL FORAMEN

1

HEAVENLY SURGE

Strengthen and calm the Spirit

SHEN SOURCE

13

Calm emotions, calm Spirit

HEAD OVERLOOKING TEARS

15

Balance emotions

Strengthen and calm the Spirit

Hui point for tendons

Clear Liver Qi stag

Relax tendons

Clear Liver Qi stag

34

YANG MOUND SPRING

Clear Channel for hip problems/sciatica

JUMPING CIRCLE

30

Hui Point for bone marrow

39

HANGING CUP

Nourish Kidney Jing and Marrow

SUN AND MOON

Front Mu of GB

Clear Clear Clear

Damp-Heat

24

Liver Qi stag

Eliminate int/ext Wind

Eliminate Liver Yang Rising

20

WIND POND

Subdue Liver Yang Rising

43

PINCHED RAVINE

Tonify Qi and Blood

4 Flowers + BL 17

19

Clear Damp-Heat from Liv and GB

37

BRIGHT AND CLEAR

Any eye problem

Junction Point

YANG SUPPORT

SEDATION

38 **38**

Subdue Liver Yang Rising or Fire

ANCESTRAL MOUND

40

Source Point

Clear Liver Qi stag

Benefit breasts by clearing Liver Qi

Dai Mai

41

FOOT OVERLOOKING TEARS

41

GB 26 Daimai Girdle Channel

Tonifying actions: Activate the Channel.

Dispersing actions: Regulate *Dai Mai* (maybe with GB 41 and TB 5). Resolve Damp-Heat in the lower *jiao*. Regulate the Uterus.

GB 30 Huantiao Jumping Circle
Meeting Point of GB and Bl

Tonifying actions: Tonify *Qi* and Blood and activate the Channel.

Dispersing actions: Remove obstructions from the Channel. Resolve Damp-Heat.

Main use: Channel problems affecting the hip or causing sciatica.

GB 31 Fengshi Wind Market

Tonifying actions: Activate the Channel.

Dispersing actions: Expel (external) Wind. Relieve itching (often with TB 6 for urticaria). Remove obstructions from the Channel. Relax tendons.

GB 34 Yanglingquan Yang Mound Spring *Earth Point, He Sea Point, Hui Point for Tendons*

Tonifying actions: Strengthen the Gall Bladder. Nourish the tendons. Activate the Channel.

Dispersing actions: Promote smooth flow of Liver *Qi*. Resolve Damp-Heat in Liver/Gall Bladder. Remove obstructions from the Channel. Relax tendons. Harmonise *Shaoyang*.

Main uses: To clear Liver *Qi* Stagnation (often with Liv 3). To clear Damp-Heat in the Liver/Gall Bladder. For tendon problems.

GB 36 Waiqiu Outer Mound *Xi-Cleft Point*

Dispersing actions: Remove obstructions from the Channel. Stop pain (Channel and Organ).

GB 37 Guangming Bright and Clear *Luo-Junction Point*

Tonifying actions: Strengthen the Spirit of the Gall Bladder.

Dispersing actions: Expel Wind. Clear Heat. Conduct Fire downwards. Brighten the eyes. Remove obstructions from the Channel.

Main uses: For any eye problems. As Junction Point to strengthen the relationship with the Liver (often with Liv 5).

GB 38 Yangfu Yang Support *Fire Point, Sedation Point, Jing-River Point*

Tonifying actions: Strengthen the Gall Bladder.

Dispersing actions: Subdue Liver *Yang*. Clear Heat. Resolve Damp-Heat in the Gall Bladder. Harmonise *Shaoyang*. Remove obstructions from the Channel.

Main uses: As the Sedation Point to treat Wood (CF, often with Liv 2). To subdue Liver *Yang* Rising or Liver Fire.

GB 39 Xuanzhong Hanging Cup
Hui Point for Bone Marrow

Tonifying actions: Strengthen *Jing*. Nourish Marrow and bone marrow. Strengthen the Bones and sinews.

Dispersing actions: Expel Wind (in Channel).

Main uses: Nourish Kidney Jing, Marrow and Bones (especially in the elderly and in chronic *Bi* syndrome). Acute stiff neck from Wind (compare with SI 3).

GB 40 Qiuxu Ancestral Mound
Yuan-Source Point

Tonifying actions: Strengthen the Spirit of the Gall Bladder. Strengthen the *Hun*.

Dispersing actions: Promote smooth flow of Liver *Qi*. Clear Heat and Damp-Heat in the Gall Bladder. Remove obstructions from the Channel. Regulate the *Shaoyang*.

Main uses: As the Source Point to strengthen Wood (CF, usually with Liv 3). Clear Liver *Qi* Stagnation. Local and distal point for Channel problems (Gall Bladder and Triple Burner).

GB 41 Zulinqi Foot Overlooking Tears *Wood Point, Horary Point, Shu-Stream Point, Exit Point, Opening Point of Dai Mai*

Tonifying actions: Strengthen the Spirit of the Gall Bladder.

Dispersing actions: Promote smooth flow of Liver *Qi*. Benefit the breasts. Subdue Liver *Yang*. Resolve Damp-Heat. Regulate *Dai Mai*.

Main uses: As the Opening Point of *Dai Mai* (usually with TB 5). Relieve Liver *Qi* stagnation affecting the breasts.

GB 43 Xiaxi Pinched Ravine *Water Point, Tonification Point, Ying-Spring Point*

Tonifying actions: Strengthen the Gall Bladder.

Dispersing actions: Subdue Liver *Yang*. Resolve Damp-Heat (in the Gall Bladder Channel). Benefit the ears.

Main uses: To subdue Liver *Yang*. As the Tonification Point to treat Wood (CF, often with Liv 8).

GB 44 Zuqiaoyin Foot Hole Yin
Jing-Well Point, Metal Point

Dispersing actions: Subdue Liver *Yang*. Clear Heat and brighten the eyes. Calm the Spirit.

Bl 19 Danshu Gall Bladder Back Shu Point

Tonifying actions: Tonify Gall Bladder *Qi*.

Dispersing actions: Subdue Liver *Yang*. Resolve Damp-Heat in the Gall Bladder and Liver. Subdue rebellious Stomach *Qi*. Relax the diaphragm. Regulate *Shaoyang*.

Main uses: To strengthen Wood CF (with Bl 18). To tonify *Qi* and Blood with Bl 17 (4 Flowers). To clear Damp-Heat from the Liver and Gall Bladder.

The Liver Channel

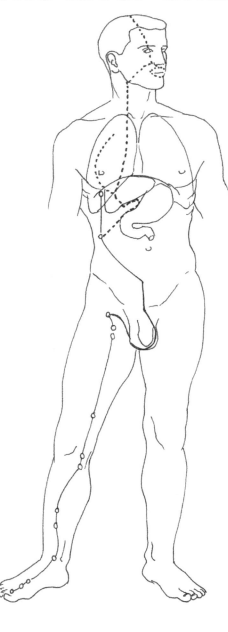

'The **Liver** holds the office of general of the armed forces. Assessment of circumstances and conception of plans stem from it.'

SU WEN CHAPTER 8

The **Wood Element** enables us to appropriately assert ourselves in the world, to have a clear vision of our own unique path in life, to have structures and boundaries in order that the path can unfold and make plans and decisions.

Physical areas particularly affected by Liver points

Anywhere on the Liver Channel, especially:

- Head and eyes

- Throat and chest

- Hypochondrium

- Abdomen

- Uterus

- External genitals and bladder

- Medial aspect of the legs

LIVER POINT FUNCTIONS (HAND JUEYIN)

Liv 1 Dadun **Great Mound** *Wood Point, Horary Point, Jing-Well Point, Entry Point*

Tonifying actions: Strengthen Liver *Qi*.

Dispersing actions: Promote smooth flow of Liver *Qi*. Regulate menstruation. Stop menstrual bleeding. Resolve Damp-Heat in the genito-urinary system. Restore consciousness.

Main use: Promote smooth flow of Liver *Qi*, especially in the lower *jiao*. Stop menstrual bleeding.

Liv 2 Xingjian **Moving Between** *Fire Point, Sedation Point, Ying-Spring Point*

Tonifying actions: Strengthen Liver *Qi* and *Yang*.

Dispersing actions: Clear Liver Fire. Subdue Liver *Yang*. Subdue Liver Wind. Cool Blood and stop bleeding. Resolve Damp-Heat in the genito-urinary system.

Main uses: To subdue Liver *Yang* Rising or Liver Fire. As Sedation Point to treat Wood CF (often with GB 38).

Liv 3 Taichong **Great Surge** *Yuan-Source Point, Earth Point, Shu-Stream Point*

Tonifying actions: Nourish Liver Blood and *Yin*. Strengthen Liver *Qi*. Strengthen the Spirit.

Dispersing actions: Promote the smooth flow of Liver *Qi*. Subdue Liver *Yang*. Subdue internal Wind. Calm the Spirit. Calm spasms.

Main uses: As the Source Point to strengthen Wood CF (usually with GB 40). For Liver *Qi* stagnation, *Yang* Rising or Blood Xu. With LI 4 as 'The Four Gates' to relieve spasm, descend *Qi* from the head and calm the mind.

Liv 4 Zhongfeng **Middle Seal** *Metal Point, Jing-River Point*

Tonifying actions: Strengthen Liver *Qi*. Strengthen the Spirit.

Dispersing actions: Promote the smooth flow of Liver *Qi* in the lower *jiao*. Resolve Damp-Heat in the genito-urinary system.

Liv 5 Ligou **Woodworm Canal** *Luo-Junction Point*

Tonifying actions: Strengthen Liver *Qi*.

Dispersing actions: Promote the smooth flow of Liver *Qi*, and treat plumstone *Qi*. Resolve Damp-Heat in the genito-urinary system.

Main uses: Treat genital and urinary problems arising from Damp-Heat. Treat *Qi* stagnation, especially affecting the throat. As the Junction Point to strengthen the relationship with the Gall Bladder (often with GB 37).

Liv 6 Zhongdu **Middle Capital** *Xi-Cleft Point*

Tonifying actions: Strengthen Liver *Qi*.

Dispersing actions: Remove obstructions from the Channel. Promote the smooth flow of Liver *Qi* and stop pain in the lower *jiao* (e.g. acute urinary pain).

Liv 8 Ququan **Crooked Spring** *Water Point, Tonification Point, He Sea Point*

Tonifying actions: Nourish Liver Blood and *Yin*. Benefit tendons.

Dispersing actions: Resolve Damp and Damp-Heat in the lower *jiao*. Benefit the Bladder and genitals. Regulate Liver *Qi* and Blood and benefit the Uterus.

Main use: To nourish Liver Blood and *Yin*. As the Tonification Point to treat Wood CF (often with GB 43). As a local point for knee problems.

Liv 10–Liv 12

Main uses: Secondary local points for Damp-Heat, Damp-Cold, stagnation of *Qi*, Blood or Cold, in the area of the upper thigh, groin, genitals, bladder and Uterus. Liv 12 in particular eliminates cold from the Liver Channel when used with moxa.

Liv 13 Zhangmen **Chapter Gate** *Front Mu Point of Sp, Hui Point for Five Yin Organs*

Tonifying actions: Tonify the Spleen (and Stomach). Strengthen the Spirit.

Dispersing actions: Promote the smooth flow of Liver *Qi*. Harmonise the Liver and Spleen. Resolve Damp-Heat in the Liver and Gall Bladder. Calm the Spirit.

Main uses: For digestive disorders arising from Liver *Qi* stagnation invading the Spleen. Treat Wood (CF) and treat the Spirit.

Liv 14 Qimen **Gate of Hope** *Front Mu Point of Liv, Exit Point, Meeting Point of Sp and Liv*

Tonifying actions: Strengthen Liver *Qi*. Strengthen the Spirit.

Dispersing actions: Promote the smooth flow of Liver *Qi* and regulate Blood in the middle and upper *jiao*. Benefit the breasts. Harmonise the Liver and Stomach. Resolve Damp-Heat in the Liver and Gall Bladder. Calm the Spirit.

Main uses: As the Exit Point (often with Lu 1). For digestive disorders arising from Liver *Qi* stagnation invading the Stomach. Treat Wood (CF) and treat the Spirit.

Bl 18 Ganshu **Liver Back Shu Point**

Tonifying actions: Strengthen Liver *Qi* and nourish Liver Blood. Benefit the sinews. Strengthen the Spirit.

Dispersing actions: Promote the smooth flow of Liver *Qi*. Regulate Blood. Clear Heat. Resolve Damp-Heat in the Liver and Gall Bladder. Subdue Liver Wind. Brighten the eyes.

Main uses: To strengthen Wood CF (with Bl 19). Often used with Bl 17 and Bl 20, 'The Magnificent Six', to nourish Blood. Treat any Liver pattern.

Bl 47 Hunmen **Hun Gate/Door of Hun**

Tonifying actions: Strengthen Liver *Qi* and root the *Hun*. Strengthen the Spirit.

Dispersing actions: Regulate Liver *Qi*.

Main use: Root the *Hun* and strengthen the Spirit.

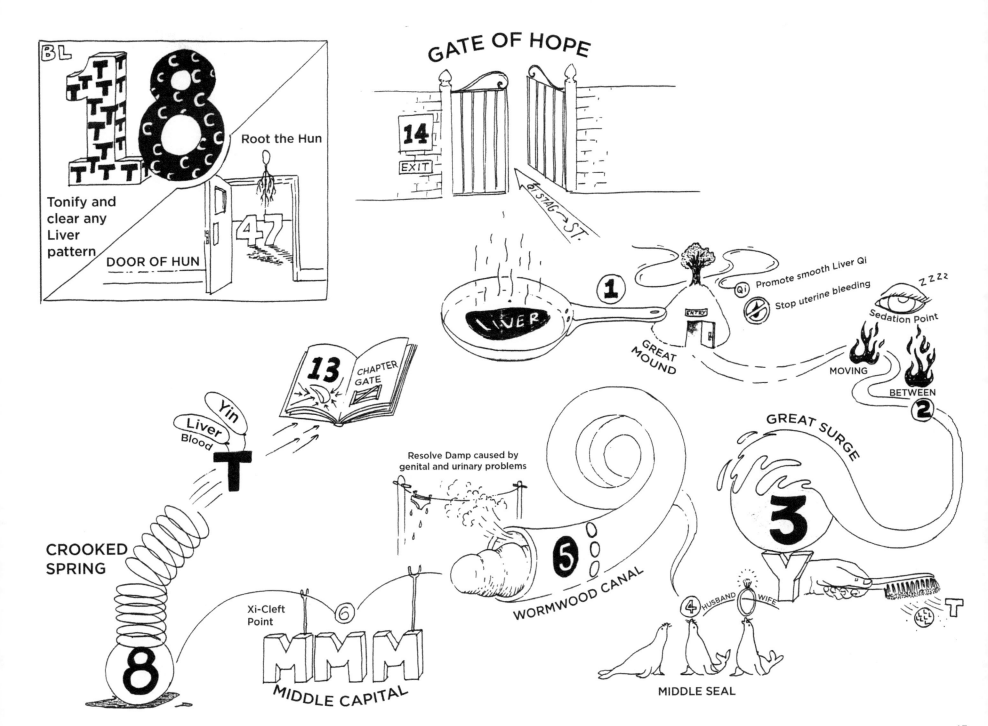

BL

18

Tonify and clear any Liver pattern

Root the Hun

DOOR OF HUN

47

GATE OF HOPE

14
EXIT

Qi STAG ST.

1
GREAT MOUND
ENTRY

Qi Promote smooth Liver Qi

Stop uterine bleeding

ZZZZ
Sedation Point

MOVING
BETWEEN
2

GREAT SURGE

13
CHAPTER GATE

Yin
Liver
Blood
T

Resolve Damp caused by genital and urinary problems

5
WORMWOOD CANAL

3
Y
T

4 HUSBAND WIFE

MIDDLE SEAL

CROOKED SPRING

8

Xi-Cleft Point

6
MMM
MIDDLE CAPITAL

Notes

The Lung Channel

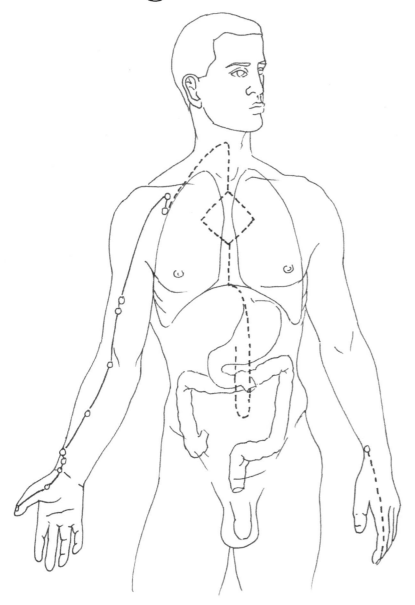

'The **Lung** holds the office of minister and chancellor. The regulation of the life-giving network stems from it.'

SU WEN CHAPTER 8

The **Metal Element** enables us to feel loss and move on, take in the richness of life, and accept that when something is over we must let go.

Physical areas particularly affected by Lung points

- Upper *jiao* (Lungs and Heart)

- Nose

- Anywhere on the Lung Channel

- Connects with the Large Intestine and Spleen Channels, which strengthen its influence on *Qi* and Blood

- Descends *Qi* and opens the Water Passages, thus influencing the Bladder and Kidneys

LUNG POINT FUNCTIONS (HAND TAIYIN)

Lu 1 Zhongfu **Central Treasury** *Entry Point, Front Mu Point of Lu*

Tonifying actions: Tonify Lung *Qi*. Strengthen the descending function of Lung *Qi*. Strengthen Spirit (Metal CF).

Dispersing actions: Disseminate and descend Lung *Qi* and stop in cough and wheezing. Resolve Phlegm and clear Heat from the Lungs. Disperse fullness in the chest and stop pain.

Main uses: Acute excess Lung patterns. Disperse fullness in the chest. As the Entry Point (often with Liv 14). Tonify Lung *Qi*, strengthen Metal (CF), treat the Spirit.

Lu 2 Yunmen **Cloud Gate**

Tonifying actions: Tonify Lung *Qi*. Strengthen the descending function of Lung *Qi*.

Dispersing actions: Disperse fullness in the chest. Clear Lung Heat. Stop cough.

Main uses: Treat Metal (CF) and treat the Spirit. Disperse fullness in the chest.

Lu 3 Tianfu **Heavenly Treasury** *Window of Heaven*

Tonifying actions: Unite Heaven and Earth. Strengthen the descending function of Lung *Qi*.

Dispersing actions: Regulate the ascending and descending of Lung *Qi*. Clear Lung Heat. Cool the Blood and stop bleeding (nose, lung). Calm the *Po*.

Main use: As the Window of Heaven (Metal CF, usually with LI 18).

Lu 5 Chize **Foot Marsh/Water Marsh** *Water Point, Sedation Point He Sea Point*

Tonifying actions: Tonify *Yin* and moisten the Lungs.

Dispersing actions: Clear Lung Heat. Resolve Phlegm from the Lung. Descend rebellious Lung *Qi*. Regulate the Water Passages and benefit the Bladder. Relax tendons (Channel).

Main uses: Clear Heat or Phlegm in the Lung. As the Sedation Point (often with LI 2).

Lu 6 Kongzui **Biggest Hole** *Xi-Cleft Point*

Tonifying actions: Tonify Lung *Qi*.

Dispersing actions: Clear Lung Heat. Stop bleeding (coughing or vomiting blood). Regulate and descend Lung *Qi*. Remove obstructions from the Channel. Moderate acute conditions of Lung (Organ or Channel).

Lu 7 Lieque **Broken Sequence** *Exit Point, Luo-Junction Point, Opening Point of Ren Mai*

Tonifying actions: Tonify Lung *Qi* and strengthen the descending and dispersing function. Circulate *Wei Qi*. Open *Ren Mai*. Communicate with the Large Intestine.

Dispersing actions: Release the Exterior and expel external Wind. Open the nose and benefit the head and neck. Regulate ascending and descending of *Qi* to and from head. Benefit the Bladder and open the Water Passages. Remove obstructions from the Channel.

Main uses: Release the Exterior and expel external pathogenic Wind and benefit the nose, head and neck (often with LI 4). Opening Point of *Ren Mai* (often with Coupled Point Kid 6). As the Junction Point to strengthen the relationship with the Large Intestine (often with LI 6). Exit point with LI 4.

Lu 8 Jingqu **Channel Ditch** *Metal Point, Horary Point, Jing-River Point*

Tonifying actions: Tonify Lung *Qi*.

Dispersing actions: Descend Lung *Qi* and alleviate cough and wheeze.

Main use: As the Horary Point to treat Metal (CF), often with LI 1.

Lu 9 Taiyuan **Great Abyss** *Earth Point, Yuan-Source Point, Tonification Point, Shu-Stream Point, Hui Point for Arteries and Blood Vessels*

Tonifying actions: Tonify Lung *Qi* and *Yin*. Tonify *Zong Qi*. Promote circulation of Blood and influence the pulse.

Dispersing actions: Resolve Phlegm. Promote descending and dispersing of Lung *Qi* and stop cough. Clear Lung and Liver Heat.

Main use: As the Source Point or Tonification Point to strengthen Metal CF (usually with LI 4 or LI 11). Tonify Lung *Qi*, Lung *Yin* and *Zong Qi*.

Lu 10 Yuji **Fish Border** *Fire Point, Ying-Spring Point*

Tonifying actions: Warm the Lungs.

Dispersing actions: Clear Lung Heat. Benefit the throat.

Main use: Clear Heat from the Lung (Organ and Channel).

Lu 11 Shaoshang **Lesser Metal** *Wood Point, Jing-Well Point*

Dispersing actions: Expel external and internal Wind. Clear Heat. Promote the descending and dispersing of Lung *Qi*. Benefit the throat. Promote resuscitation.

Main use: Acute sore throat from external pathogenic Wind-Heat (can be bled).

Bl 13 Feishu **Lung Back Shu Point**

Tonifying actions: Tonify Lung *Qi* and *Yin*.

Dispersing actions: Promote the descending and dispersing function of Lung *Qi*. Release the Exterior. Regulate *Ying* and *Wei Qi*. Clear Lung Heat.

Main use: Strengthen Metal CF (usually with Bl 25). To treat any Lung syndrome – external or internal, excess or deficient.

Bl 42 Pohu **Door of Po**

Tonifying actions: Tonify Lung *Qi*, strengthen the *Po*.

Dispersing actions: Promote the descending and dispersing of Lung *Qi*. Soothe breathlessness and alleviate cough. Clear obstructions from the Channel (chest, back, neck).

Main uses: Strengthen and support the *Po*. Strengthen Metal (CF). Treat the Spirit.

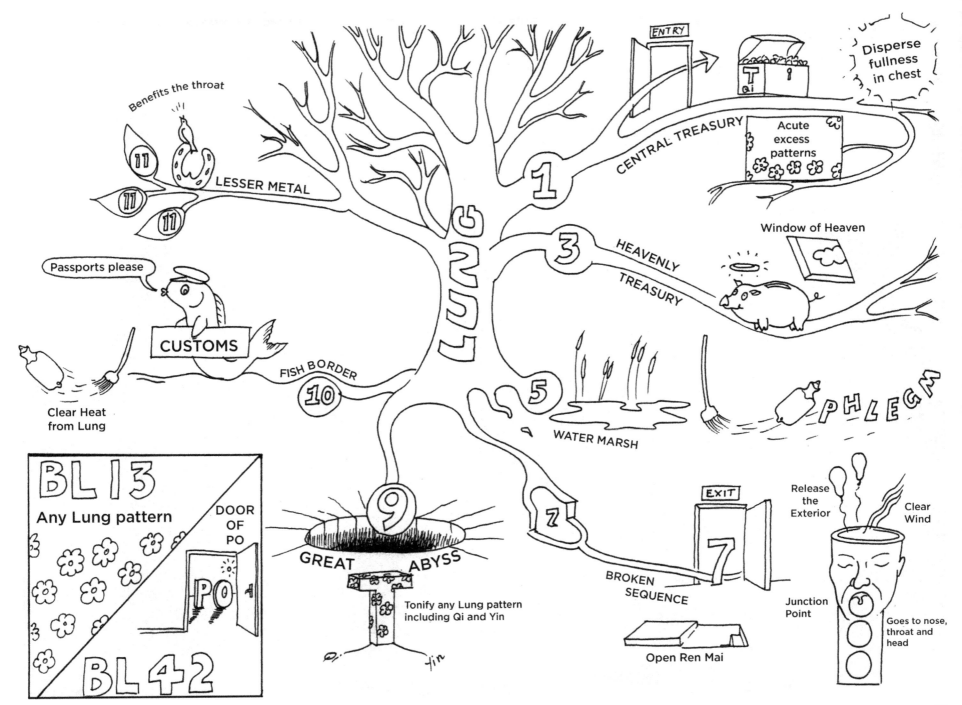

Notes

The Large Intestine Channel

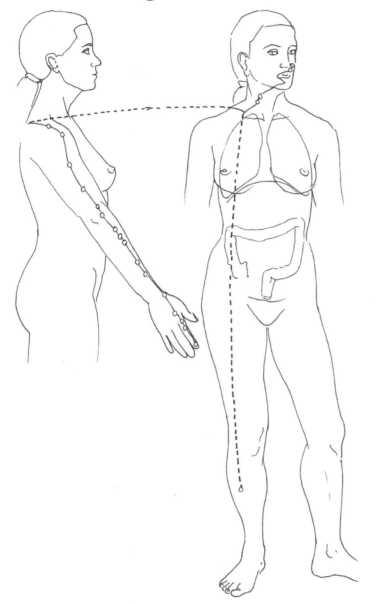

'The **Large Intestine** is responsible for transit. The residue from transformation stems from it.'

SU WEN CHAPTER 8

The **Metal Element** enables us to feel loss and move on, take in the richness of life, and accept that when something is over we must let go.

Physical areas particularly affected by Large Intestine points

- Head, face, nose, teeth, neck, shoulder and arm

- Stomach and Intestines

- Connects with the Small Intestine and Bladder Channels and the *Yang Qiao Mai*, which strengthens its influence on the shoulder and neck

- Connects with the Lung – some points assist Lung functions

LARGE INTESTINE POINT FUNCTIONS (HAND YANGMING)

LI 1 Shangyang **Metal Yang** *Metal Point, Horary Point, Jing-Well Point*

Tonifying actions: Tonify the Large Intestine.

Dispersing actions: Clear Heat (fevers, eyes, throat). Calm the Spirit. Expel Wind and scatter Cold. Extinguish internal Wind and promote resuscitation. Remove obstructions from the Channel (local and distal).

Main uses: Clear Heat in the Large Intestine. As the Horary Point to strengthen Metal (CF, usually with Lu 8).

LI 2 Erjian **Second Interval** *Water Point, Sedation Point (often with Lu 5), Ying-Spring Point*

Tonifying actions: Cool and bring fluids/fluidity to the Large Intestine (Organ and Channel).

Dispersing actions: Clear Heat (Channel and Organ). Remove obstructions from the Channel (local and distal).

LI 3 Sanjian **Third Interval** *Wood Point, Shu-Stream Point*

Dispersing actions: Expel EP Wind and Heat. Brighten the eyes, benefit the throat (acute Wind Heat). Expel Wind and Cold from the Channel (*Bi* syndrome of the hand).

LI 4 Hegu **Joining Valley** *Yuan-Source Point, Entry Point*

Tonifying actions: Tonify *Qi* and consolidate the Exterior. Promote labour.

Dispersing actions: Expel external pathogenic Wind. Release the Exterior. Regulate *Wei Qi* and sweating. Harmonise the ascending and descending of *Qi*. Relax muscular tension. Calm the mind. Remove obstructions from the Channel.

Main uses: As the Source Point to strengthen Metal CF (usually with Lu 9). Tonify *Qi*. Expel Wind-Cold (with e.g. Lu 7) and Wind-Heat (with e.g. TB 5). Benefit the face. With Liv 3 as 'The Four Gates' to relieve spasm, bring *Qi* down from the head and calm the mind.

LI 5 Yangxi **Yang Stream** *Fire Point, Jing-River Point*

Tonifying actions: Tonify and warm Large Intestine *Qi*.

Dispersing actions: Expel external pathogenic Wind. Release the Exterior. Clear Heat (*Yangming* fevers) and thus calm the Spirit. Benefit the wrist joint.

LI 6 Pianli **Slanting Passage** *Luo-Junction Point*

Tonifying actions: Communicate with the Lung.

Dispersing actions: Open the Water Passages. Remove obstructions from the Channel (local point).

Main uses: Open Lung Water Passages. As the Junction Point to strengthen the relationship with the Lung (often with Lu 7).

LI 7 Wenliu **Warm Flow** *Xi-Cleft Point*

Tonifying actions: Can be used with Lu 6 to strengthen Lung and Large Intestine functions. Warm Large Intestine in Metal (CF).

Dispersing actions: Clear *Yangming* Fire and thus calm the Spirit. Moderate acute conditions of the Large Intestine (Organ or Channel). Stop pain.

LI 10 Shousanli **Arm Three Miles**

Tonifying actions: Tonify *Qi* (Channel and Organ; maybe with St 36).

Dispersing actions: Remove obstructions from the Channel.

LI 11 Quchi **Crooked Pond** *Earth Point, Tonification Point, He Sea Point*

Tonifying actions: Tonify *Qi* of the Large Intestine (Organ and Channel).

Dispersing actions: Clear Heat (acute and chronic). Cool Blood. Expel Wind (especially when moving from external to internal). Relieve itching. Resolve Damp. Remove obstructions from the Channel.

Main uses: As the Tonification Point to strengthen Metal CF (usually with Lu 9). Clear Heat and/or Damp. Cool Blood. Helpful for skin disorders.

LI 14 Binao **Upper Arm's Musculature** *Meeting Point of LI, SI and BI, Point of Yang Wei Qiao Mai*

Tonifying actions: Strengthen *Qi* of the Channel.

Dispersing actions: Remove obstructions from the Channel. Benefit the eyes. Resolve Phlegm and dissipate nodules (neck and throat).

LI 15 Jianyu **Shoulder Joint** *Meeting Point of LI and Yang Qiao Mai*

Tonifying actions: Strengthen *Qi* of the Channel.

Dispersing actions: Remove obstructions from the Channel, expel Wind and Damp. Resolve Phlegm and dissipate nodules (neck and throat).

Main use: Shoulder problems (chronic and acute), *Shi* and *Xu*.

LI 16 Jugu **Clavicle** *Meeting Point of LI and Yang Qiao Mai*

Tonifying actions: Strengthen *Qi* of the Channel.

Dispersing actions: Remove obstructions from the Channel. Resolve Phlegm and dissipate nodules (neck and throat).

LI 18 Futu **Support the Prominence** *Window of Heaven*

Tonifying actions: Unite Heaven and Earth.

Dispersing actions: Subdue rebellious *Qi* and alleviate cough and wheezing. Resolve Phlegm and dissipate nodules. Benefit the throat and voice.

Main use: As the Window of Heaven (Metal CF, usually with Lu 3).

LI 20 Yingxiang **Welcome Fragrance** *Exit Point, Meeting Point of St and LI*

Tonifying actions: Lift the Spirit (Metal CF).

Dispersing actions: Expel Exterior Wind. Open the nose.

Main uses: As the Exit Point (often with St 1). Local point for the nose.

BI 25 *Dachangshu* **Large Intestine Back Shu Point**

Tonifying actions: Strengthen function of the Large Intestine. Strengthen the lower back.

Dispersing actions: Remove obstructions from the Channel (Bladder Channel – low back). Regulate *Qi* of the Large Intestine and alleviate pain.

Main uses: Strengthen Metal (CF, usually with Bl 13). Treat any Large Intestine syndrome. Local point for low back problems.

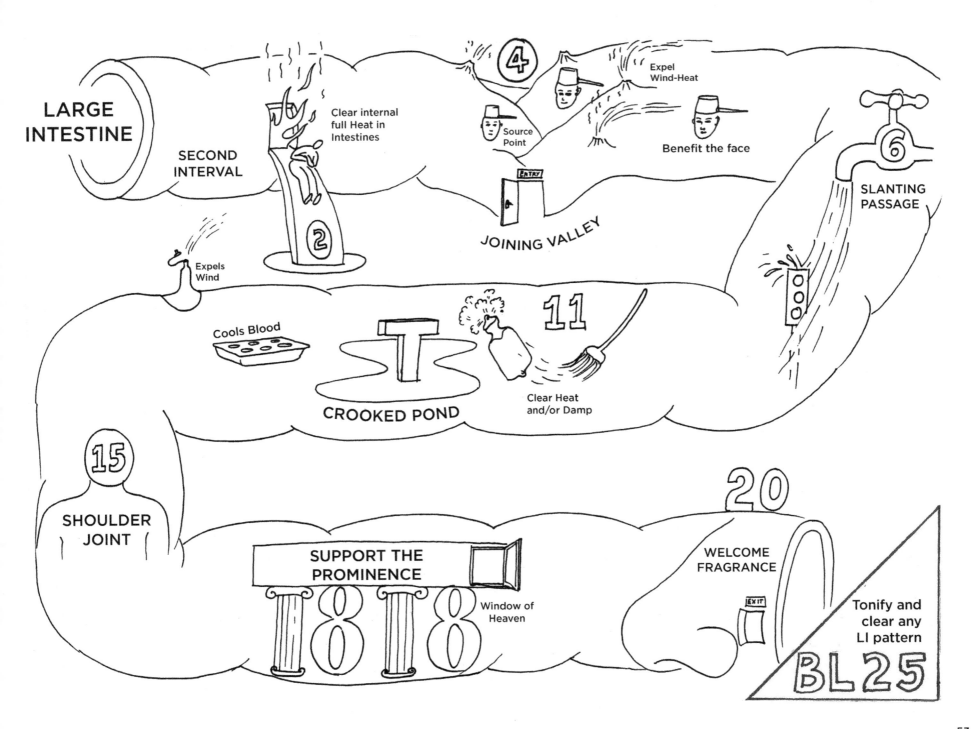

Notes

The Stomach Channel

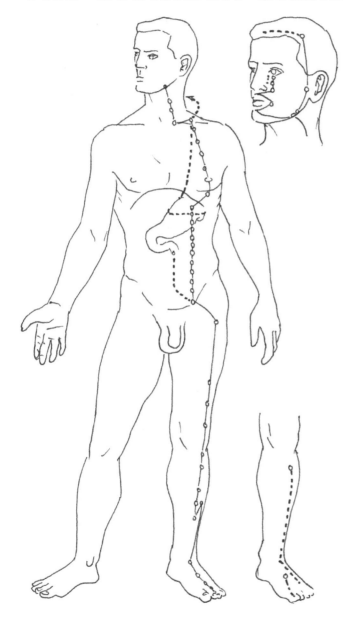

'The **Spleen and Stomach** are responsible for the storehouses and granaries. The five tastes stem from them.'

SU WEN CHAPTER 8

The **Earth Element** enables us to give support and nourishment to others, ask for help and take in nurture and care when it is offered to us, and distinguish between when it is appropriate to look after our needs and when to care for others.

Physical areas particularly affected by Stomach points

- Anywhere on the Stomach Channel

- Middle and lower *jiao* (digestive organs and bowels)

- Connects with the Large Intestine, which strengthens its influence on bowel function

- Connects with the Gall Bladder, which aids its influence on digestion and on the eyes and ears

- Rebellious Stomach *Qi* can affect the Heart and upper *jiao*

STOMACH POINT FUNCTIONS (FOOT YANGMING)

St 1 Chengqi **Receive Tears** *Entry Point*

Tonifying actions: To open Entry Point in entry-exit block.

Dispersing actions: Expel Wind (internal and external). Stop lacrimation. Clear Heat. Benefit the eyes.

Main uses: As the Entry Point (often with LI 20). Local point for eye problems.

St 2 Sibai **Four Whites**

Dispersing actions: Expel Wind (internal and external). Stop lacrimation. Clear Heat. Benefit the eyes.

Main use: Local point for eye and sinus problems.

St 3 Juliao **Great Foramen**

Tonifying actions: Activate the Channel.

Dispersing actions: Expel Wind (from face). Dissipate swelling. Remove obstructions from the Channel.

Main use: Local point for problems of the face, nose or eyes.

St 4 Dicang **Earth Granary** *Meeting Point of St and LI*

Tonifying actions: Strengthen Earth (nourishing function).

Dispersing actions: Expel Wind (from face). Remove obstructions from the Channel.

Main uses: Local point for deviation of the mouth or eye. Strengthen Earth (CF).

St 6 Jiache **Jaw Chariot**

Tonifying actions: Activate the Channel.

Dispersing actions: Expel Wind (from face). Remove obstructions from the Channel (face/neck/teeth/jaw).

St 7 Xiaguan **Below the Joint** *Meeting Point of St and GB*

Tonifying actions: Activate the Channel.

Dispersing actions: Remove obstructions from the Channel. Expel Wind. Benefit the ears, jaw and teeth.

St 8 Touwei **Corner of the Head** *Meeting Point of St and GB*

Dispersing actions: Expel Wind (internal or external). Relieve pain. Benefit the eyes. Clear the head. Relieve dizziness.

Main use: Clear the head, especially of Damp, Phlegm or Wind.

St 9 Renying **People Welcome** *Window of Heaven. Meeting Point of St and GB Point of the Sea of Qi (with Ren 17, Bl 10)*

Tonifying actions: Unite Heaven and Earth (Earth CF). Tonify *Qi* (with Ren 17 and Bl 10).

Dispersing actions: Regulate ascending and descending of *Qi*. Subdue rebellious *Qi*. Relieve swelling (throat and neck).

Main uses: As the Window of Heaven (Earth CF). Regulate Blood pressure.

St 12 Quepen **Empty Basin**

Tonifying actions: Strengthen Earth (CF). Activate the Channel.

Dispersing actions: Subdue Rebellious *Qi* (chest). Remove obstructions from the Channel (local).

St 13–St 16

Tonifying actions: Activate the Channel.

Dispersing actions: Descend rebellious *Qi* (chest).

St 14 Kufang **Storehouse**

Tonifying actions: Strengthen the Spirit (Earth CF).

Dispersing actions: Descend rebellious *Qi* (chest).

St 18 Rugen **Breast Root**

Tonifying actions: Activate the Channel.

Dispersing actions: Benefit the breast and reduce swelling. Facilitate lactation. Move *Qi* in the chest and stop cough.

St 20 Chengman **Receiving Fullness**

Tonifying actions: Strengthen the Spirit (Earth CF).

Dispersing actions: Harmonise middle *jiao*. Subdue rebellious *Qi* (Stomach and Lung).

St 21 Liangmen **Beam Gate**

Tonifying actions: Raise *Qi* and stop diarrhoea.

Dispersing actions: Move Stomach *Qi* and stop pain. Clear Stomach Heat.

Main use: Acute Stomach problems.

St 25 Tianshu **Heavenly Pivot** *Front Mu Point of LI, Point to Release Internal Dragons*

Tonifying actions: Tonify and strengthen the Spirit (Earth CF). Promote function of the Large Intestine.

Dispersing actions: Clear Heat (in Stomach and Intestines – *Yangming* fevers). Regulate *Qi* and Blood in lower *jiao*. Resolve Damp and Damp-Heat (Intestines and oedema). Relieve retention of food. Calm the Spirit. Release Internal Dragons.

Main uses: Promote function of the Large Intestine in any intestinal problem (deficient or excess). Clear Damp-Heat in the lower *jiao* (often with St 36 or St 37). Tonify *Qi* of the lower *jiao*. Tonify and strengthen the Spirit (Earth CF). Release Internal Dragons (with Ren 15, St 32, St 41).

St 27 Daju **Great Fullness**

Tonifying actions: Benefit the Kidneys and support the *Jing*.

Dispersing actions: Regulate *Qi* of the Intestines. Resolve Damp and promote urination.

Main use: Acute lower *jiao* problems.

St 28 Shuidao **Water Way**

Tonifying actions: Tonify and raise *Qi* in lower *jiao*.

Dispersing actions: Regulate *Qi*, Blood and fluids in lower *jiao*. Regulate menstruation. Open the Water Passages and benefit urination. Stop pain.

Main uses: Urinary retention. Stagnation of *Qi*, Blood or fluids in menstrual and other gynaecological problems.

St 29 Guilai **Returning**

Tonifying actions: Warm lower *jiao*. Tonify and raise *Qi* of lower *jiao*.

Dispersing actions: Move Blood stasis. Warm Cold in lower *jiao* (with moxa).

Main use: Menstrual problems from stagnation of Blood and/or Cold.

St 30 Qichong **Surging Qi** *Point of Chong Mai, Point of Sea of Food*

Tonifying actions: Tonify *Jing*. Tonify pre- and post-Heavenly *Qi*. Raise *Qi*.

Dispersing actions: Regulate *Chong Mai*. Regulate *Qi* in lower *jiao*. Subdue rebellious Stomach *Qi*. Regulate Blood in the Uterus.

Main use: Tonify pre- and post-Heavenly *Qi*.

 Continued on page 58

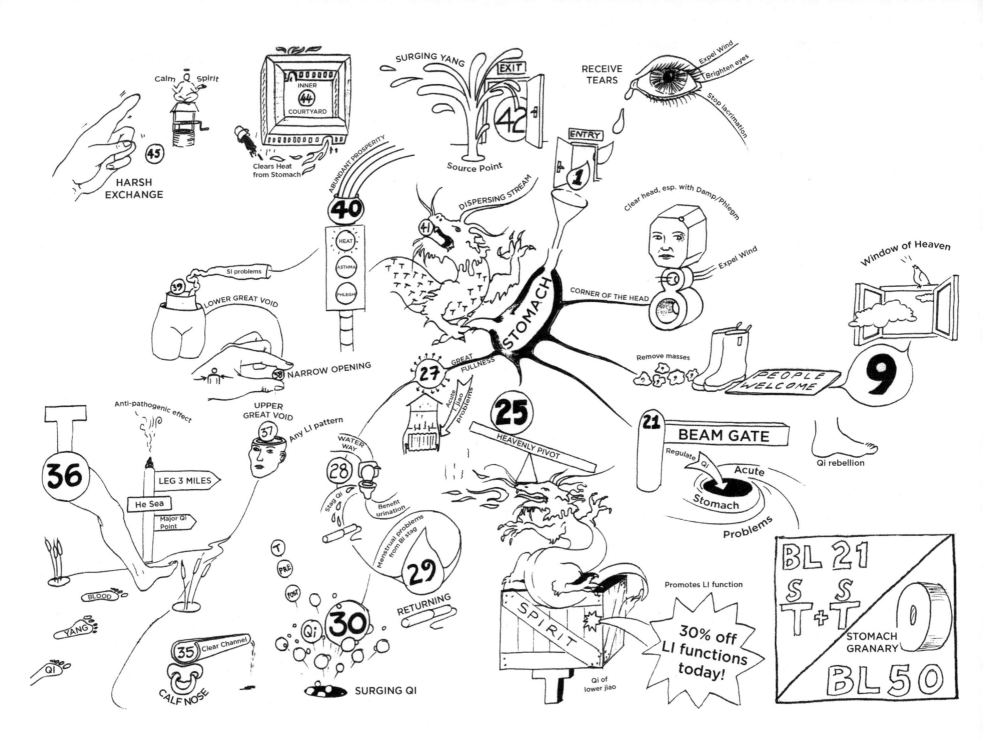

57

St 31 Biguan **Thigh Gate**

Tonifying actions: Tonify *Qi* in the Channel (*Wei* syndrome).

Dispersing actions: Remove obstructions from the Channel. Expel Wind and Damp (*Bi* and *Wei* syndromes).

St 32 Futu **Prostrate Hare** *Point to Release Internal Dragons*

Tonifying actions: Activate the Channel.

Dispersing actions: Remove obstructions from the Channel. Expel Wind and Damp (*Bi* and *Wei* syndromes). Release Internal Dragons.

Main use: Release Internal Dragons (with Ren 15, St 25, St 41).

St 34 Liangqiu **Beam Mound** *Xi-Cleft Point*

Tonifying actions: Activate the Channel.

Dispersing actions: Subdue Rebellious Stomach *Qi*. Remove obstructions from the Channel. Expel Damp, Wind and Cold (*Bi* syndrome).

Main uses: Acute disorders of the Stomach. *Bi* syndrome of the knee.

St 35 Dubi **Calf Nose**

Dispersing actions: Remove obstructions from the Channel. Relieve swelling. Stop pain.

Main use: *Bi* syndrome of the knee (often used with *Xiyan* Extra Point: 'Eyes of the Knee').

St 36 Zusanli **Leg 3 Miles** *Earth Point, Horary Point, He Sea Point, Point of Sea of Food*

Tonifying actions: Strengthen the Stomach and Spleen (and thus clear Damp). Tonify *Qi* and Blood. Raise *Yang*. Revive *Yang* and restore consciousness. Nourish Stomach *Yin*. Support and harmonise *Ying* and *Wei Qi*.

Dispersing actions: Regulate the Intestines. Harmonise the Stomach. Expel Wind, Damp and Cold. Resolve oedema. Remove obstructions from the Channel.

Main uses: As the Horary Point to treat Earth (CF, often with Sp 3). Major point to strengthen *Qi*, *Yang* (often with Ren 6) and Blood. Use moxa for anti-pathogenic effect and to strengthen resistance to disease. Any Stomach problem (deficient or excess). *Bi* syndrome of the knee.

St 37 Shangjuxu **Upper Great Void** *Lower He Sea Point of LI, Point of Sea of Blood*

Dispersing actions: Regulate the Stomach and Intestines. Eliminate Damp-Heat (in the Large Intestine). Resolve retention of food. Remove obstructions from the Channel.

Main use: As the Lower He Sea Point of the Large Intestine for chronic and acute problems of the Large Intestine.

St 38 Tiaokou **Narrow Opening**

Tonifying actions: Activate the Channel.

Dispersing actions: Remove obstructions from the Channel. Expel Wind and Damp (*Bi*). Benefit the shoulder (empirical).

Main use: Acute shoulder problems.

St 39 Xiajuxu **Lower Great Void** *Lower He Sea Point of SI, Point of Sea of Blood*

Tonifying actions: (Rarely used but can tonify Blood.)

Dispersing actions: Move Small Intestine *Qi* and transform stagnation. Regulate the Intestines and clear Damp-Heat. Remove obstructions from the Channel. Eliminate Wind-Damp (*Bi* and *Wei* syndromes).

Main use: For acute Small Intestine problems.

St 40 Fenglong **Abundant Prosperity** *Luo-Junction Point*

Tonifying actions: Tonify Stomach and strengthen Earth (CF).

Dispersing actions: Resolve Phlegm and Damp. Calm and clear the Spirit. Open the chest. Promote descending of Lung *Qi*. Remove obstructions from the Channel.

Main uses: Clear Phlegm. As the Junction Point to strengthen the relationship with the Spleen (often with Sp 4).

St 41 Jiexi **Dispersing Stream** *Fire Point, Tonification Point, Jing-River Point, Point to Release Internal Dragons*

Tonifying actions: Tonify Stomach *Qi*.

Dispersing actions: Clear (Stomach) Heat. Calm the Spirit. Remove obstructions from the Channel.

Main uses: As the Tonification Point to strengthen Earth (CF, often with Sp 2). Release Internal Dragons (with Ren 15, St 25, St 32).

St 42 Chongyang **Surging** *Yang Yuan-Source Point, Exit Point*

Tonifying actions: Tonify the Stomach and Spleen.

Dispersing actions: Harmonise the Stomach. Calm the Spirit. Remove obstructions and clear Heat from the Channel.

Main uses: As the Source Point to strengthen Earth (CF, usually with Sp 3). Tonify the Stomach.

St 43 Xiangu **Sinking Valley** *Wood Point, Shu-Stream Point*

Tonifying actions: Activate the Channel.

Dispersing actions: Eliminate Wind and Heat (*Bi*). Remove obstructions from the Channel. Regulate the Stomach and Intestines.

St 44 Neiting **Inner Courtyard** *Water Point, Ying-Spring Point*

Dispersing actions: Clear Heat (Stomach Organ and Channel). Regulate Intestines and resolve Damp-Heat. Stop pain. Promote digestion. Expel Wind from the face.

Main uses: Clear Heat from the Stomach. Clear Heat Wind from the Stomach Channel (often with LI 4).

St 45 Lidui **Harsh Exchange** *Metal Point, Sedation Point, Jing-Well Point*

Dispersing actions: Clear Heat (Stomach Organ and Channel). Calm the Spirit. Brighten the eyes. Relieve Retention of food.

Main use: As the Sedation Point to calm Earth (CF, usually with Sp 5). Calm the Spirit.

Bl 21 Weishu **Stomach Back Shu Point**

Tonifying actions: Tonify Stomach *Qi*.

Main use: Strengthen Earth CF (usually with Bl 20). Tonify the Stomach and Spleen.

Bl 50 Weicang **Stomach Granary**

Tonifying actions: Tonify Stomach *Qi* and strengthen the Spirit.

Dispersing actions: Harmonise middle *jiao*.

Main use: Strengthen the Spirit (Earth CF) often with Bl 49 or Bl 21.

The Spleen Channel

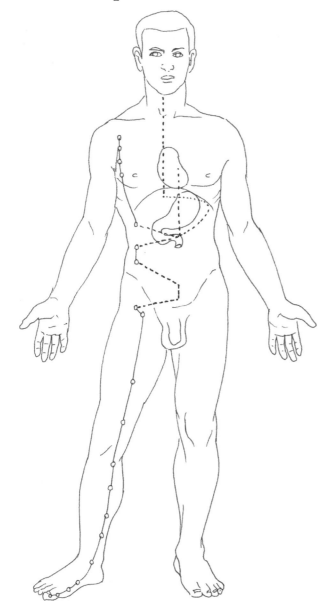

'The **Spleen and Stomach** are responsible for the storehouses and granaries. The five tastes stem from them.'

SU WEN CHAPTER 8

The **Earth Element** enables us to give support and nourishment to others, ask for help and take in nurture and care when it is offered to us, and distinguish between when it is appropriate to look after our needs and when to care for others.

Physical areas particularly affected by Spleen points

- Middle and lower *jiao* (digestive tract, Uterus, bladder and bowel)

- The chest

- The four limbs

- Anywhere on the Channel

- Connects with the Liver, Kidney and *Ren* Channels, which strengthens its influence on Blood, the Uterus and the Bladder

- Connects with the Stomach Channel, which assists its influence on digestion

- Connects with the Heart Channel and can therefore influence the Heart and chest

SPLEEN POINT FUNCTIONS (FOOT TAIYIN)

Sp 1 Yinbai **Hidden White** *Wood Point, Jing-Well Point, Entry Point*

Tonifying actions: Strengthen the Spleen. Stop bleeding. Strengthen the Spirit.

Dispersing actions: Regulate the Spleen. Regulate Blood. Calm the Heart and Spirit and restore consciousness.

Main use: Strengthen the Spleen function of holding Blood, especially for uterine bleeding. Moxa often used.

Sp 2 Dadu **Great Capital** *Fire Point, Tonification Point, Ying-Spring Point*

Tonifying actions: Strengthen the Spleen. Promote digestion.

Dispersing actions: Harmonise the middle *jiao*. Clear Heat. Resolve Damp and Damp-Heat.

Main uses: As the Tonification Point to strengthen Earth CF (usually with St 41). Clear Heat (i.e. fevers) affecting middle and lower *jiao*.

Sp 3 Taibai **Greater White** *Earth Point, Yuan-Source Point, Horary Point, Shu-Stream Point*

Tonifying actions: Strengthen the Spleen and the *Yi*. Strengthen the spinal muscles (often with Du 20 or Kidney points).

Dispersing actions: Resolve Damp and Damp-Heat. Harmonise Spleen and Stomach.

Main uses: As the Source (or Horary) Point to strengthen Earth (CF, usually with St 42 or St 36). Tonify Spleen *Qi* and Spleen *Yang*. Resolve Damp.

Sp 4 Gongsun **Grandfather and Grandson** *Luo-Junction Point, Opening Point of Chong Mai (Coupled Point of Yin Wei Mai)*

Tonifying actions: Tonify the Stomach and Spleen.

Dispersing actions: Regulate *Chong Mai*. Regulate menstruation. Stop bleeding. Move *Qi* and Blood. Harmonise middle *jiao* and dispel fullness. Benefit the Heart and chest. Calm the Spirit.

Main uses: As the Junction Point to strengthen the relationship with the Stomach (often with St 40). As the Opening Point of *Chong Mai* (often with Coupled Point Pc 6).

Sp 5 Shangqiu **Metal Mound** *Metal Point, Sedation Point, Jing-River Point*

Tonifying actions: Strengthen the Stomach and Spleen.

Dispersing actions: Regulate Damp. Benefit sinews and joints. Calm Earth (CF, often with St 45).

Sp 6 Sanyinjiao **Three** *Yin* **Meeting** *Meeting Point of Three Yin Channels of the Leg*

Tonifying actions: Strengthen the Spleen. Tonify the Kidney. Nourish *Yin* and Blood. Strengthen the Spirit.

Dispersing actions: Resolve Damp. Promote Liver function and smooth flow of *Qi*. Benefit urination. Regulate the Uterus and menstruation. Induce labour. Move Blood and eliminate stasis. Cool Blood. Stop pain. Calm the Spirit.

Main uses: Tonify *Qi*, Blood, *Yin* or *Yang*. Resolve Damp (often with Sp 9). Disharmonies of the lower *jiao*.

Sp 8 Diji **Earth Movement** *Xi-Cleft Point*

Tonifying actions: Strengthen the Spleen. Tonify *Qi* and Blood.

Dispersing actions: Regulate *Qi* and Blood. Regulate the Uterus and menstruation. Stop pain, stop bleeding. Remove obstructions from the Channel.

Main use: Acute period pain.

Sp 9 Yinlingquan *Yin* **Mound Spring** *Water Point, He Sea Point*

Tonifying actions: (Rarely used, but can strengthen the Spleen and moisturise Earth.)

Dispersing actions: Resolve Damp. Benefit the lower *jiao*. Open the Water Passages and benefit urination. Remove obstructions from the Channel.

Main uses: Resolve Damp (often with Sp 6). Benefit the lower *jiao*. Knee problems.

Sp 10 Xuehai **Sea of Blood**

Tonifying actions: Nourish Blood.

Dispersing actions: Cool Blood. Remove Blood Stasis. Regulate menstruation.

Main use: For Blood – cool, move and nourish Blood.

Sp 12 Chongmen **Surging Gate** *Meeting Point of Sp and Liv*

Dispersing actions: Remove obstructions from the Channel. Regulate *Qi* and Blood. Subdue rebellious *Qi* in *Chong Mai*. Resolve Damp and benefit urination.

Main use: Abdominal fullness and pain.

Sp 13 Fushe **Treasury Dwelling**;
Sp 14 Fijjie **Abdomen Knot**

Dispersing actions: Regulate *Qi*. Alleviate pain. Subdue rebellious *Qi* (lower *jiao*).

Sp 15 Daheng **Great Horizontal**

Tonifying actions: Strengthen the Spleen. Strengthen the limbs. Promote Large Intestine function. Strengthen the Spirit (Earth CF).

Dispersing actions: Resolve Damp. Regulate *Qi*. Stop pain.

Main uses: Promote Large Intestine function; diarrhoea or constipation (deficient or excess). Tonify *Qi* of the lower *jiao* (often with Ren 6 or St 36). Strengthen the Spirit (possibly with St 25)

Sp 18 Tianxi **Heavenly Stream**

Tonifying actions: Strengthen the Spirit. Benefit the breast and promote lactation.

Dispersing actions: Regulate and descend *Qi* (chest). Benefit the breast and promote lactation. Calm the Spirit.

Main uses: Strengthen the Spirit (Earth CF). Calm the Spirit. Breast abcess. Lactation problems.

Continued on page 62

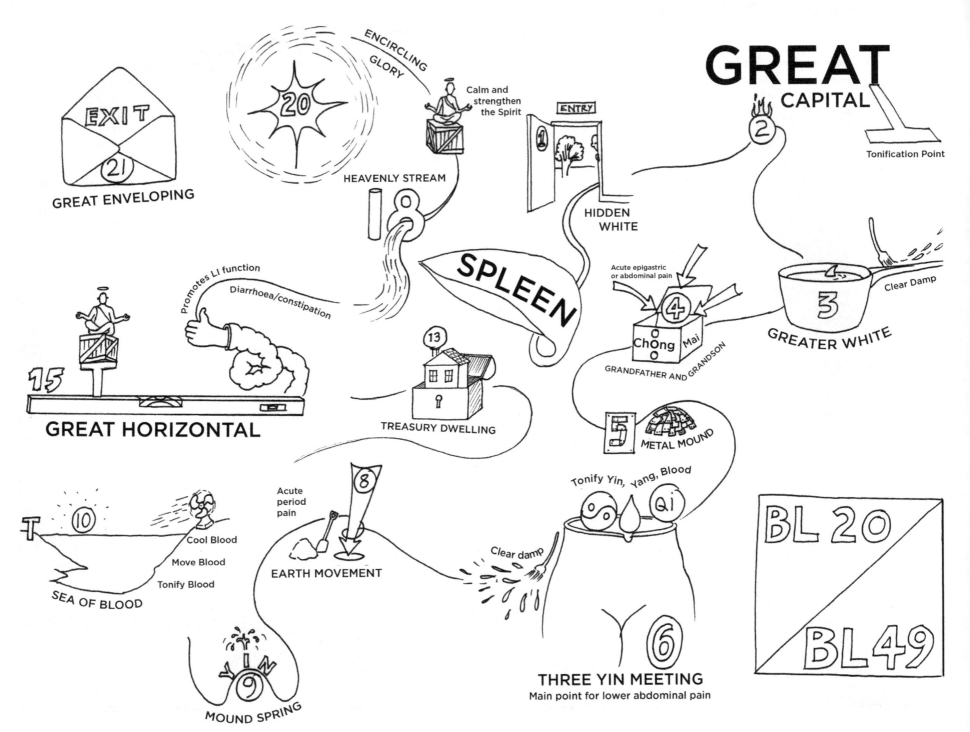

GREAT ENVELOPING

ENCIRCLING GLORY

Calm and strengthen the Spirit

HEAVENLY STREAM

GREAT CAPITAL

Tonification Point

HIDDEN WHITE

ENTRY

SPLEEN

Acute epigastric or abdominal pain

Chong Mai

GRANDFATHER AND GRANDSON

GREATER WHITE

Clear Damp

Promotes LI function

Diarrhoea/constipation

GREAT HORIZONTAL

TREASURY DWELLING

METAL MOUND

Tonify Yin, Yang, Blood

Qi

Cool Blood
Move Blood
Tonify Blood

SEA OF BLOOD

Acute period pain

EARTH MOVEMENT

Clear damp

THREE YIN MEETING
Main point for lower abdominal pain

MOUND SPRING

BL 20

BL 49

Sp 20 Zhourong **Encircling Glory**

Tonifying actions: Strengthen the Spirit.

Dispersing actions: Regulate and descend *Qi* (chest). Calm the Spirit.

Main use: Strengthen the Spirit (Earth CF). Calm the Spirit.

Sp 21 Dabao **Great Enveloping** *Exit Point, General Luo-Junction Point*

Tonifying actions: Strengthen the Spirit.

Dispersing actions: Move Blood in the Blood *Luo* Channels. Regulate *Qi* in the chest.

Main uses: Strengthen the Spirit (Earth CF). As the Exit Point (often with He 1). Pain in whole body (from Blood stasis in *Luo* Channels).

Bl 20 Pishu **Spleen Back Shu Point**

Tonifying actions: Tonify the Spleen and Stomach. Nourish Blood.

Dispersing actions: Resolve Damp.

Main uses: Strengthen Earth CF (with Bl 21). Tonify the Spleen and Stomach. Nourish Blood (with Bl 17 and Bl 18, 'The Magnificent Six', or with Bl 23).

Bl 49 Yishe **Yi Dwelling**

Tonifying actions: Tonify the Spleen. Stimulate memory and concentration. Strengthen the Spirit, benefit the *Yi*.

Main use: Strengthen the Spirit (Earth CF), benefit the *Yi*.

The Du Channel

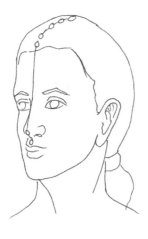

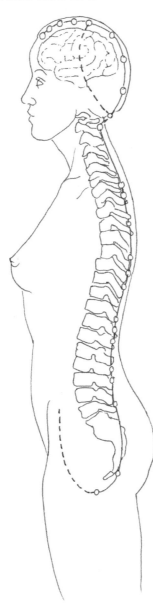

'For all the *yang* functions inside the body it is the administrative centre…[the **Du Mai**] is where all the *yang qi* is mastered… Another name for the *Du Mai* is the sea of the *yang mai*.'

ELISABETH ROCHA DE LA VALLEE, *THE EIGHT EXTRAORDINARY MERIDIANS*, P.26

The **Du Mai** influences the whole of the back of the body. It is also called the sea of the *Yang* Channels.

Physical areas particularly affected by Du points

- Spine, head and brain

- Anus, rectum, genitals and Intestines

- Bladder and Kidneys

- Heart

- Connects with the Bladder Channel, and some points assist Bladder function

- Connects with the *Ren Mai* and promotes the balance between the *Ren Mai* and *Du Mai*

DU POINT FUNCTIONS

Du 1 Changqiang Long Strength *Entry Point, Luo-Junction Point of Du*

Tonifying actions: Strengthen the spine, especially lumbar/sacral spine. Strengthen the Spirit.

Dispersing actions: Regulate the *Du* and *Ren Mai*. Resolve Damp and Damp-Heat. Regulate the two lower orifices. Subdue internal Wind. Calm the Spirit. Remove obstructions from the Channel.

Main uses: Local point for haemorrhoids and prolapsed anus. Entry Point (with Du 28, Ren 1 and Ren 24).

Du 2 Yaoshu Lumbar Shu

Tonifying actions: Strengthen the lower back.

Dispersing actions: Subdue internal Wind. Calm spasms and convulsions.

Du 3 Yaoyangguan Lumber Yang Joint *(Level with Bl 25)*

Tonifying actions: Strengthen the lower back and legs. Tonify (Kidney) *Yang*.

Dispersing actions: Dispel Wind and Damp. Remove obstructions from the Channel and ease stiffness.

Main use: Local point for lower back problems, especially if due to Kidney *Yang* Xu (e.g. with Du 5).

Du 4 Mingmen Gate of Life *(Level with Bl 23 and Bl 52)*

Tonifying actions: Tonify and warm Kidney *Yang*. Warm *Mingmen*/the Gate of Life. Tonify *Yuan Qi*. Nourish *Jing*, clear and support the *Shen*. Strengthen the spine and lower back.

Dispersing actions: Expel internal Cold (from *Yang Xu*). Regulate *Du Mai*.

Main use: Tonify Kidney *Yang* and *Yuan Qi*. Warm *Mingmen* (with moxa). (NB Du 4 is a very warming point so avoid moxa if there are any signs of Heat.)

Du 5 Xuanshu Suspended Pivot *(Level with Bl 22 and Bl 51)*

Tonifying actions: Strengthen the spine and lower back (often used with Du 3).

Dispersing actions: Remove obstructions from the Channel and ease stiffness.

Du 8 Jinsuo Contracted Tendon *(Level with Bl 18 and Bl 47)*

Tonifying actions: Strengthen the muscles and spine.

Dispersing actions: Soothe the Liver. Subdue internal Wind. Relax the tendons. Relieve spasm. Calm the Spirit (especially nervous tension affecting middle and lower *jiao*).

Main use: To relax spasm and contraction of the back muscles. Ease rigidity of body, mind or Spirit (usually for Wood CF).

Du 9 Zhiyang Reaching Yang *(Level with Bl 17)*

Tonifying actions: Strengthen the Spleen. Strengthen the back.

Dispersing actions: Regulate the Liver and Gall Bladder. Resolve Damp and Damp-Heat. Regulate the middle *jiao*. Move *Qi*. Open the chest and diaphragm.

Main use: Treatment of jaundice, Damp-Heat in the Liver and Gall Bladder.

Du 10 Lingtai Spirit Tower

Tonifying actions: Strengthen and calm the Spirit.

Dispersing actions: Alleviate cough and wheezing. Clear Fire-poison (empirical point for furuncles and clove sores).

Main use: Strengthen and calm the Spirit (often with or before Du 11).

Du 11 Shendao Shen Way *(Level with Bl 15 and Bl 44. Similar level to Ren 17)*

Tonifying actions: Strengthen and calm the Spirit. Tonify the Heart and Lung.

Dispersing actions: Regulate the Heart. Clear Heat and subdue internal Wind.

Main use: Strengthen and calm the Spirit (often with or after Du 10).

Du 12 Shenzhu Body Pillar *(Level with Bl 13 and Bl 42)*

Tonifying actions: Strengthen the body and spine. Strengthen the Spirit. Tonify Lung *Qi*.

Dispersing actions: Clear Heat from the Lung and Heart. Move stagnant Lung *Qi*. Subdue internal Wind. Calm back spasms.

Main use: Tonify Lung *Qi* (usually with Bl 13). Strengthen the Spirit and the body (e.g. with Bl 42 or Bl 43). Useful if depleted by chronic illness.

Du 13 Taodao Kiln Way *Meeting Point of Du and Bl (Level with Bl 11)*

Tonifying actions: Strengthen *Du Mai* in the upper back.

Dispersing actions: Clear Heat (lingering residual pathogen). Regulate *Shaoyang* (e.g. with TB 5).

Du 14 Dazhui Great Hammer *Meeting Point of Du Mai with all the Yang Channels, Point of the Sea of Qi*

Tonifying actions: Tonify *Qi* and *Yang*. Firm the Exterior.

Dispersing actions: Clear Heat. Release the Exterior and expel Wind and firm the Exterior. Regulate *Ying* and *Wei Qi*. Subdue internal Wind. Regulate the flow of *Qi* between body and neck/head, and between arms, shoulders and neck. Clear and calm the Spirit.

Main use: Clear *Yang* pathogens. Tonify *Yang* (with moxa). Neck and shoulder problems.

Du 15 Yamen Gate to Dumbness *Point of the Sea of Qi*

Tonifying actions: Restore the *Yang* to the upper orifices. Benefit the tongue and stimulate speech. Nourish the Brain and clear the mind and Spirit. Benefit the neck and spine.

Dispersing actions: Subdue internal Wind. Benefit the tongue and stimulate speech. Benefit the neck and spine.

Continued on page 66

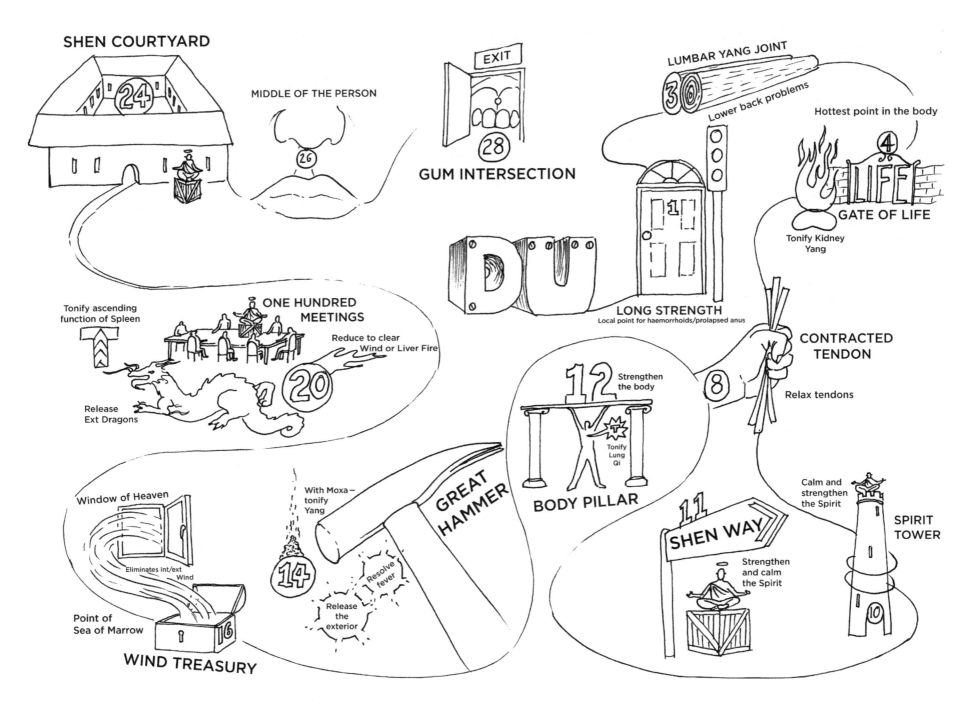

Du 16 Fengfu **Wind Treasury** *Window of Heaven Point of Sea of Marrow*

Tonifying actions: Unite the *Qi* of Heaven and Earth. Nourish Marrow and benefit the brain. Clear the Spirit.

Dispersing actions: Eliminate Wind (internal and external). Calm the Spirit.

Main use: Eliminate internal or external Wind. Window of Heaven (maybe with Ren 22).

Du 17 Naohu **Brain Door** *Meeting Point of Du and Bl*

Dispersing actions: Subdue internal Wind and benefit the brain. Calm and clear the Spirit.

Du 19 Houding **Posterior Vertex**

Tonifying actions: Can be used (often with Du 20) to unify the Zang Fu and re-establish order.

Dispersing actions: Calm the Spirit (e.g. with Ren 15 or Du 20). Subdue *Yang*. Expel Wind from the Channel.

Du 20 Baihui **One Hundred Meetings** *Meeting Point of all Yang Channels, Point of Sea of Marrow (with Du 16), Point to Release External Dragons*

Tonifying actions: Strengthen and lift the Spirit. Raise and tonify *Yang*. Nourish Marrow. Benefit the brain.

Dispersing actions: Subdue *Yang*. Calm the Spirit. Subdue internal Wind. Promote resuscitation.

Main uses: Strengthen the ascending function of *Yang* and treat prolapses. Strengthen and lift the Spirit. Reduce to eliminate Wind and clear Liver Fire. Calm the Spirit (e.g. with Du 19). Release External Dragons (with Bl 11, Bl 23 and Bl 61).

Du 23 Shangxing **Upper Star**

Dispersing actions: Open the nose (main use). Benefit the eyes.

Du 24 Shenting **Shen Courtyard** *Meeting Point of Du and St*

Tonifying actions: Strengthen and lift the Spirit.

Dispersing actions: Calm the Spirit. Subdue internal Wind. Benefit the nose and eyes.

Main uses: Calm the Spirit (e.g. with GB 13 or *Yintang*). (used in psychiatric practice for schizophrenia). Strengthen and lift the Spirit.

Du 26 Renzhong (Shuigou) **Middle of the Person (Water Drain)** *Meeting Point Du, LI and St*

Tonifying actions: Restore the connection of *Yin* with *Yang*. Restore consciousness.

Dispersing actions: Promote resuscitation. Restore consciousness. Benefit the lumbar spine. Subdue internal Wind. Expel Wind from the face and nose.

Main use: Promote resuscitation and restore consciousness (e.g. windstroke, fainting, shock). Distal point for acute lumbar sprain.

Du 28 Yinjiao **Gum Intersection** *Exit Point*

Dispersing actions: Clear Heat and benefit the gums.

Main use: Exit Point (with Du 1, Ren 1 and Ren 24).

Note: To open *Du Mai* use the Opening and Coupled Points SI 3 and Bl 62.

The Ren Channel

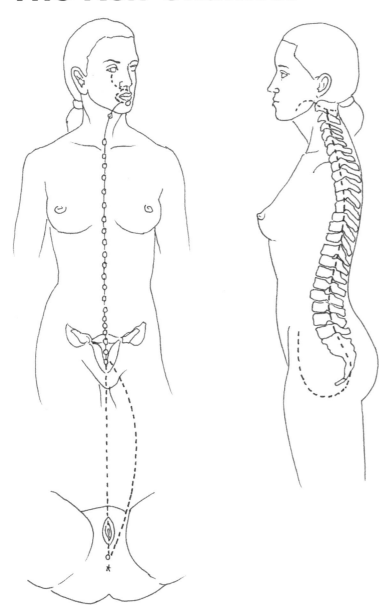

'The **Ren Mai** is…the commander and controller of all the yin functions within the body… It is called the sea of the yin meridians and the special master for the Uterus and the function of gestation within a woman.'

ELISABETH ROCHA DE LA VALLEE, *THE EIGHT EXTRAORDINARY MERIDIANS*, P.87

The **Ren Mai** influences the whole of the front of the body. It is also called the sea of the *Yin* Channels.

Physical areas particularly affected by Ren points

- Genitals, Bladder and Uterus

- Intestines, Stomach and abdomen

- Chest (Heart and Lung), throat and face

- Connects with the *Du Mai* and promotes the balance between the *Du Mai* and *Ren Mai*, and the front and the back

REN POINT FUNCTIONS

Ren 1 Huiyin Meeting of Yin *Entry Point of Ren Mai, Meeting Point of Ren, Du and Chong Mai*

Tonifying actions: Nourish *Yin*. Nourish *Jing*. Revive and calm the Spirit.

Dispersing actions: Resolve Damp and Damp-Heat. Calm the Spirit and open the orifices of the Mind. Promote resuscitation and revive from drowning.

Main uses: Entry Point (with Ren 24, Du 1 and Du 28). Local point for anal and genito-urinary problems.

Ren 3 Zhongji Middle Extremity *Front Mu Point, Meeting Point of Ren, Sp, Liv and Kid*

Tonifying actions: Tonify *Qi* of the Bladder and Kidneys, nourish *Jing* and *Yuan Qi*.

Dispersing actions: Resolve Damp and Damp-Heat and dispel stagnation in the lower *jiao*. Benefit the Uterus and regulate menstruation.

Main use: For genito-urinary problems, especially Damp-Heat in the Bladder.

Ren 4 Guanyuan Gate to the Yuan Qi *Front Mu Point of SI, Meeting Point of Ren, Sp, Liv and Kid, Meeting Point of Ren Mai and Chong Mai*

Tonifying actions: Tonify all forms of *Qi*, i.e. *Qi*, *Yang* (with moxa), Blood, *Yin*, *Jing*, *Yuan Qi*, Kidney *Yin* and *Yang*, *Wei Qi* and *Ying Qi*. Root the *Shen* and the *Hun*. Strengthen the Uterus and regulate menstruation. Benefit the Bladder.

Dispersing actions: Subdue rebellious *Qi* in *Chong Mai*. Regulate the Small Intestine (though rarely used clinically for this).

Main use: Tonifying as above, especially to nourish deficiency of *Jing*, Blood or *Yin*.

Ren 5 Shimen Stone Door *Front Mu Point of TB*

Tonifying actions: Strengthen the *Yuan Qi*. Tonify the Kidneys. Promote the transformation and excretion of fluids in the lower *jiao*.

Dispersing actions: Open the Water Passages. Regulate the transformation of fluids in the lower *jiao*. Regulate the lower *jiao*. Regulate the Uterus.

Ren 6 Qihai Sea of Qi

Tonifying actions: Tonify *Qi* and *Yang*. Raise sinking *Qi*. Tonify *Yuan Qi*.

Dispersing actions: Regulate *Qi* and Blood. Resolve Damp.

Main uses: Tonify *Qi* and *Yang* (e.g. with St 36, and often with moxa). Regulate *Qi* or Blood in lower *jiao* (e.g. with GB 34 or Sp 6/8/10).

Ren 7 Yinjiao Yin Crossing *Meeting Point of Ren Mai, Chong Mai and Kidneys*

Tonifying actions: Nourish *Yin*. Tonify the Kidneys.

Dispersing actions: Regulate the Uterus and menstruation. Resolve Damp from lower *jiao*.

Ren 8 Shenque Shen Palace Gate

Tonifying actions: Warm *Yang* and rescue collapse. Strengthen the Spleen and Kidney *Yang*. Tonify *Yuan Qi*. Strengthen the Spirit.

Main uses: (Moxa only, on a bed of salt.) Warm and stabilise *Yang*. Strengthen the Spirit. To treat chronic or acute diarrhoea from Cold.

Ren 9 Shuifen Water Separation

Tonifying actions: Promote the transformation of fluids.

Dispersing actions: Regulate the Water Passages. Harmonise the Intestines and dispel accumulation (of food, fluids or *Qi*).

Main use: Resolve Damp in the middle and lower *jiao*. Treat oedema and ascites.

Ren 10 Xiawan Lower Epigastrium *Meeting Point of Ren and Sp*

Tonifying actions: Promote descending of Stomach *Qi*. Tonify the Stomach and Spleen.

Dispersing actions: Harmonise the Stomach and dispel stagnation of food.

Main use: Descend Stomach *Qi*.

Ren 11 Jianli Established Mile

Tonifying actions: Promote the Stomach function of rotting and ripening. Promote descending of Stomach *Qi*.

Dispersing actions: Harmonise the middle *jiao* and regulate *Qi* (used mainly for *Shi* conditions).

Ren 12 Zhongwan Middle Epigastrium *Front Mu Point of St, Hui Point for Yang Organs, Front Mu Point of Middle Jiao, Meeting Point of Ren Mai, SI, TB and St*

Tonifying actions: Tonify the Stomach and Spleen. Resolve Damp (by tonifying the functions of transformation and transportation). Strengthen and calm the Spirit (worry, anxiety, etc.).

Dispersing actions: Subdue rebellious Stomach *Qi*. Regulate Stomach *Qi*.

Main uses: Tonify the Stomach and Spleen for digestive problems, especially from deficiency. Strengthen and calm the Spirit. Resolve Damp (anywhere).

Ren 13 Shangwan Upper Epigastrium

Dispersing actions: Subdue rebellious Stomach *Qi*. Harmonise the Stomach. Can also regulate the Heart and calm the Spirit.

Main use: Subdue rebellious Stomach *Qi*, especially in acute patterns. Treat hiccups. Can treat morning sickness in early pregnancy (with St 36 and Pc 6).

Ren 14 Juque Greatest Palace Gate *Front Mu Point of He*

Tonifying actions: Strengthen Heart *Qi*. Strengthen the Spirit.

Dispersing actions: Regulate Heart *Qi* (and thus calm the Spirit). Transform Phlegm. Clear Heat from the Heart. Harmonise the Stomach and subdue rebellious Stomach *Qi*.

Main use: Tonify the Heart. Treat Fire (CF) and treat the Spirit. Clear Heart Fire or Phlegm (e.g. with He 8 or Pc 5).

Continued on page 70

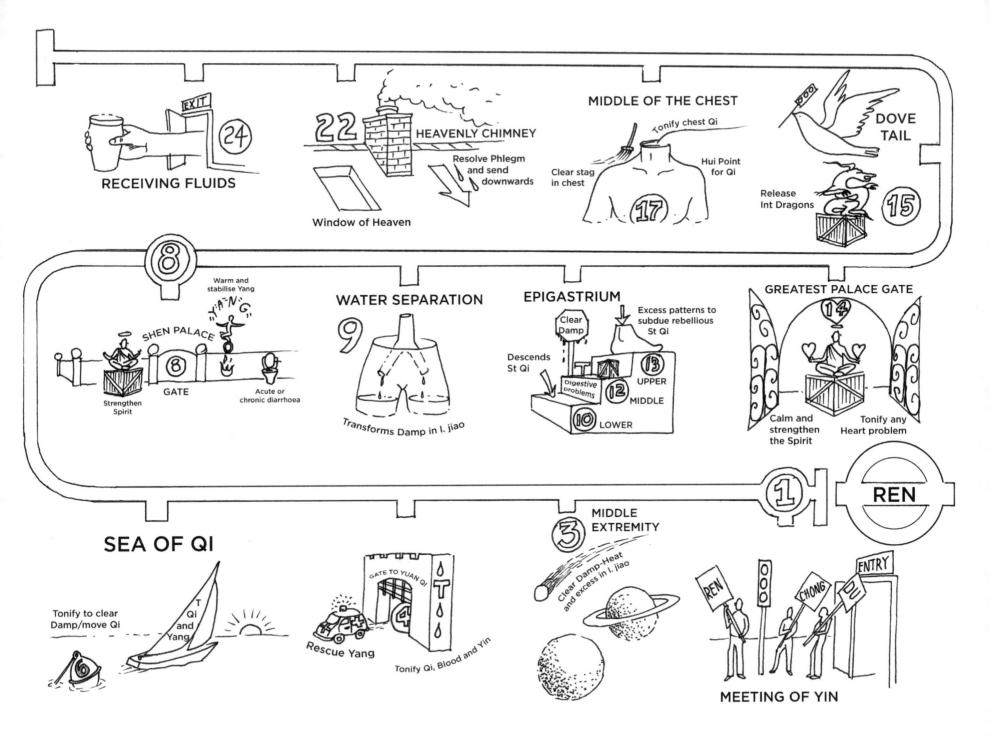

EXIT

24

RECEIVING FLUIDS

22

HEAVENLY CHIMNEY

Resolve Phlegm and send downwards

Window of Heaven

MIDDLE OF THE CHEST

Tonify chest Qi

Clear stag in chest

Hui Point for Qi

17

DOVE TAIL

Release Int Dragons

15

8

Warm and stabilise Yang

YANG

SHEN PALACE

8

GATE

Strengthen Spirit

Acute or chronic diarrhoea

WATER SEPARATION

9

Transforms Damp in l. jiao

EPIGASTRIUM

Clear Damp

Excess patterns to subdue rebellious St Qi

Descends St Qi

13 UPPER

Digestive problems

12 MIDDLE

10 LOWER

GREATEST PALACE GATE

14

Calm and strengthen the Spirit

Tonify any Heart problem

1

REN

SEA OF QI

Tonify to clear Damp/move Qi

6

Qi and Yang

GATE TO YUAN QI

Rescue Yang

4

Tonify Qi, Blood and Yin

3 MIDDLE EXTREMITY

Clear Damp-Heat and excess in l. jiao

REN

CHONG

ENTRY

MEETING OF YIN

Ren 15 Jiuwei **Dove Tail** *Luo-Junction Point of Ren Mai, Yuan-Source Point of Five Yin Organs, Point to Release Internal Dragons*

Tonifying actions: Strengthen the *Qi* of the Heart and Heart Protector. Nourish the *Yin* organs and thus strengthen and calm the Spirit.

Dispersing actions: Regulate Heart *Qi* (and thus calm the Spirit). Open the chest and promote the descending of Lung *Qi*.

Main use: Strengthen the Spirit. Calm the Spirit (e.g. with Du 19). Release Internal Dragons (with St 25, St 32, St 41). Open the chest (e.g. with Pc 6 or Pc 4).

Ren 17 Shanzhong **Middle of the Chest** *Front Mu Point of Pc and Upper Jiao, Hui Point for Qi, Point of the Sea of Qi (with St 9, Bl 10)*

Tonifying actions: Tonify the *Qi* of Heart Protector and Heart, and *Zong Qi*. Strengthen the Spirit.

Dispersing actions: Regulate Heart *Qi* (and thus calm the Spirit). Open the chest. Benefit breasts and promote lactation. Descend rebellious *Qi* of Lung and Stomach.

Main use: Tonify the Heart Protector and Heart. Treat Fire (CF) and treat the Spirit. Open the chest (e.g. with Pc 6 or Pc 4).

Ren 18 Yutang **Jade Hall**
Ren 19 Zigong **Purple Palace**
Ren 20 Huagai **Magnificent Canopy**

These points are not emphasised in the textbooks, but consider the significance of their names and location for treating the *Qi* of the chest, the residence of the Heart and Lung.

Ren 22 Tiantu **Heavenly Chimney**
Window of Heaven, Meeting Point of Ren Mai and Yin Wei Mai

Tonifying actions: Unite the *Qi* of Heaven and Earth. Moisten the throat and voice.

Dispersing actions: Descend rebellious *Qi* (Lung or Stomach). Resolve Phlegm. Benefit the throat and voice.

Main uses: Window of Heaven (maybe with Du 16), to augment CF treatment for any CF. Resolve Phlegm and send it downwards. Moisturise the throat and voice.

Ren 23 Lianquan **Corner Spring** *Meeting Point of Ren Mai and Yin Wei Mai*

Tonifying actions: Moisten the tongue.

Dispersing actions: Benefit the tongue and promote speech (including aphasia from windstroke, and ulcers from Heart or Small Intestine Fire). Descend rebellious Lung *Qi*.

Ren 24 Chengjiang **Receiving Fluid** *Exit Point*

Tonifying actions: Promote fluids in the mouth.

Dispersing actions: Eliminate internal Wind and remove obstructions from the Channel in the face. Regulate the *Ren Mai* (locally, and as distal point for the lower *jiao*).

Main uses: Local point for problems caused by Wind, or fluid imbalances. Exit Point (with Ren 1, Du 1 and Du 28).

Note: To open *Ren Mai*, use the Opening and Coupled Points Lu 7 and Kid 6.

Penetrating Vessel (Chong Mai)

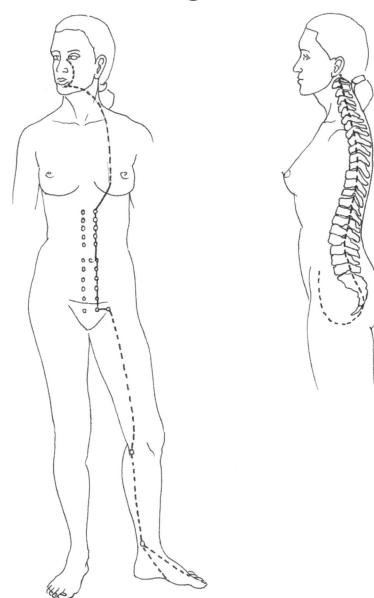

Areas influenced: Big toes, feet, medial aspect of legs, Uterus, lumbar spine, abdomen, chest, heart, breasts, throat, face and head.

Channels influenced: Spleen, Stomach, Liver, Kidneys, Heart, Small Intestine and Large Intestine.

CHANNEL FUNCTIONS
Sp 4 *Opening Point*
Pc 6 *Coupled Point*

- Move rebellious *Qi* and stagnation in chest and abdomen
- Resolve Blood stagnation in Uterus
- Nourish Blood
- Link pre- and post-Heavenly *Qi*
- Move stagnant Blood in the Heart

PENETRATING VESSEL

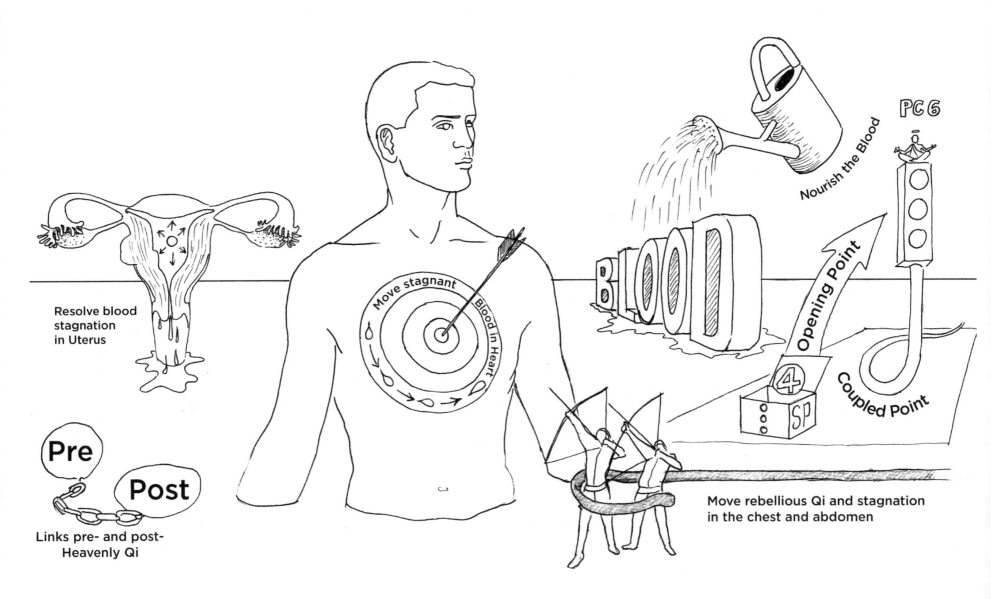

Resolve blood stagnation in Uterus

Move stagnant

Blood in Heart

Nourish the Blood

PC 6

BLOOD

Opening Point

Coupled Point

SP 4

Pre

Post

Links pre- and post-Heavenly Qi

Move rebellious Qi and stagnation in the chest and abdomen

Notes

Girdle Vessel (Dai Mai)

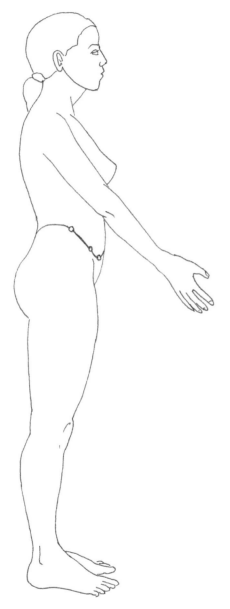

Areas influenced: Genitals, waist, hips, Uterus and bladder.

Channels influenced: Gall Bladder, Liver, Kidney (Divergent), Spleen, Stomach and Bladder.

CHANNEL FUNCTIONS
GB 41 *Opening Point*
TB 5 *Coupled Point*

- Harmonise the Liver and Gall Bladder

- Resolve Damp in the Lower Burner

- Regulate circulation of *Qi* in the legs

- Affect circulation of *Qi* in the Stomach Channel on the legs

- Influence the hip

GIRDLE VESSEL

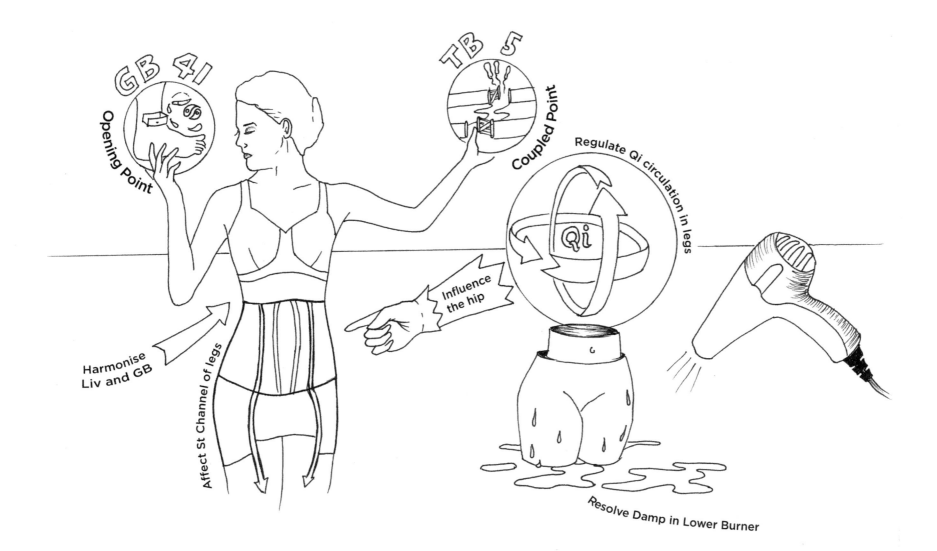

GB 41
Opening Point

TB 5
Coupled Point

Harmonise Liv and GB

Affect St Channel of legs

Influence the hip

Regulate Qi circulation in legs

Qi

Resolve Damp in Lower Burner

77

Notes

Yin Heel Vessel (Yin Qiao Mai)

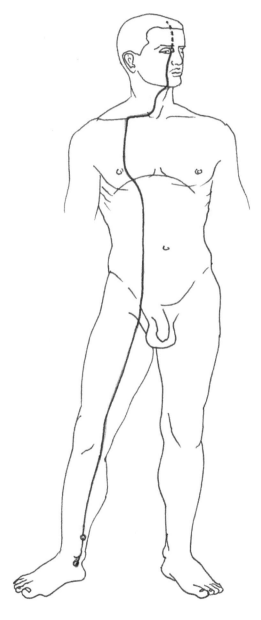

Areas influenced: Inner side of the legs, external genitalia, abdomen, eyes and brain.

Channels influenced: Kidney, Bladder and Stomach.

CHANNEL FUNCTIONS
Kid 6 *Opening Point*
Lu 7 *Coupled Point*

- Use in sleep disturbances

- Affect inner leg in *Wei* syndrome

- Clear excess patterns in the Lower Burner, which are causing unilateral symptoms

- Harmonise left and right sides

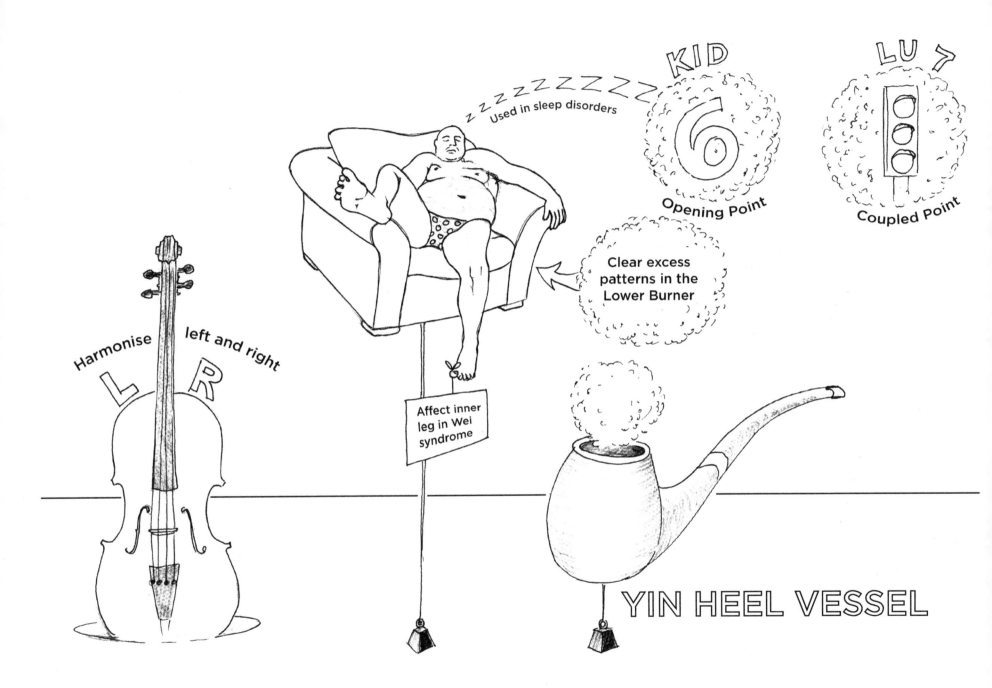

YIN HEEL VESSEL

Notes

Yang Heel Vessel (Yang Qiao Mai)

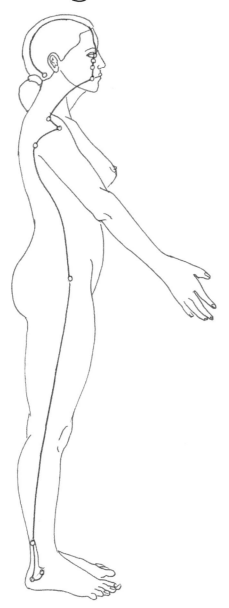

Areas influenced: Lateral aspect of feet and legs, hip, back, neck, head, eyes and brain.

Channels influenced: Bladder, Gall Bladder, Small Intestine, Large Intestine, Stomach and Triple Burner.

CHANNEL FUNCTIONS
B1 62 *Opening Point*
SI 3 *Coupled Point*

- Absorb *Yang* energy from Head

- Expel Exterior Wind

- Affect lower back and hip

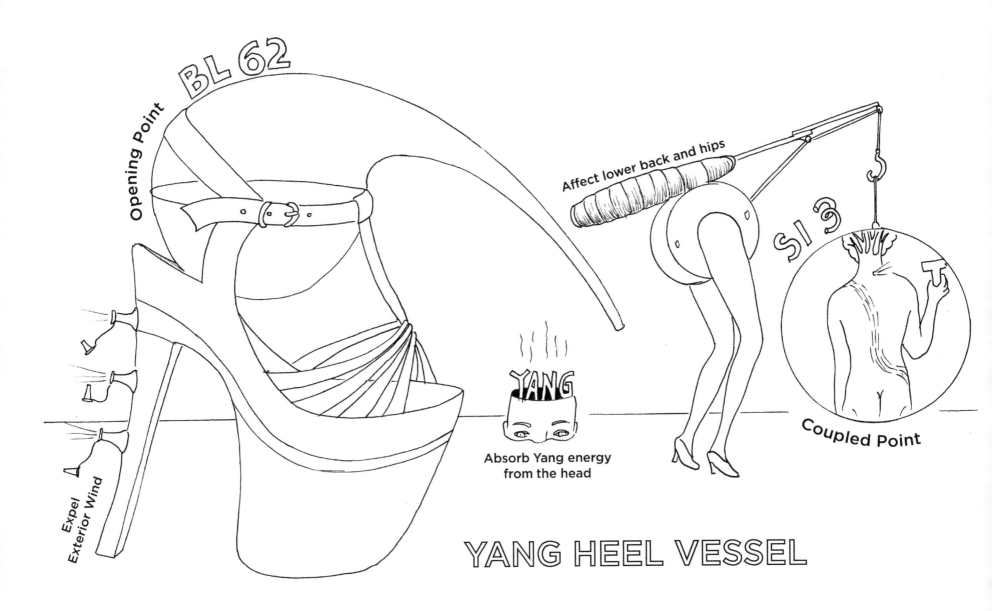

Opening Point BL 62

Expel Exterior Wind

Absorb Yang energy from the head

Affect lower back and hips

SI 3

Coupled Point

YANG HEEL VESSEL

Notes

Yin Linking Vessel (Yin Wei Mai)

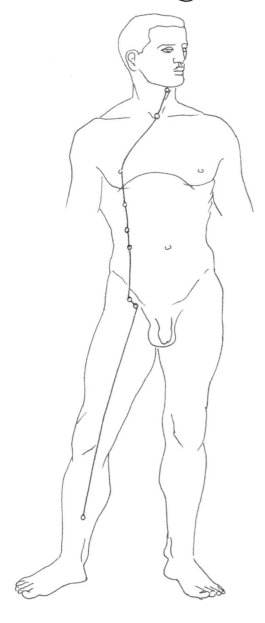

Areas influenced: Chest and heart.

Channels influenced: Heart, Pericardium, Spleen, Liver, Kidneys, Stomach and Directing Vessel.

CHANNEL FUNCTIONS

Pc 6 *Opening Point*
Sp 4 *Coupled Point*

- Nourish Blood and *Yin*

- Treat mental–emotional problems from Heart Blood deficiency

- Treat headache from Blood deficiency

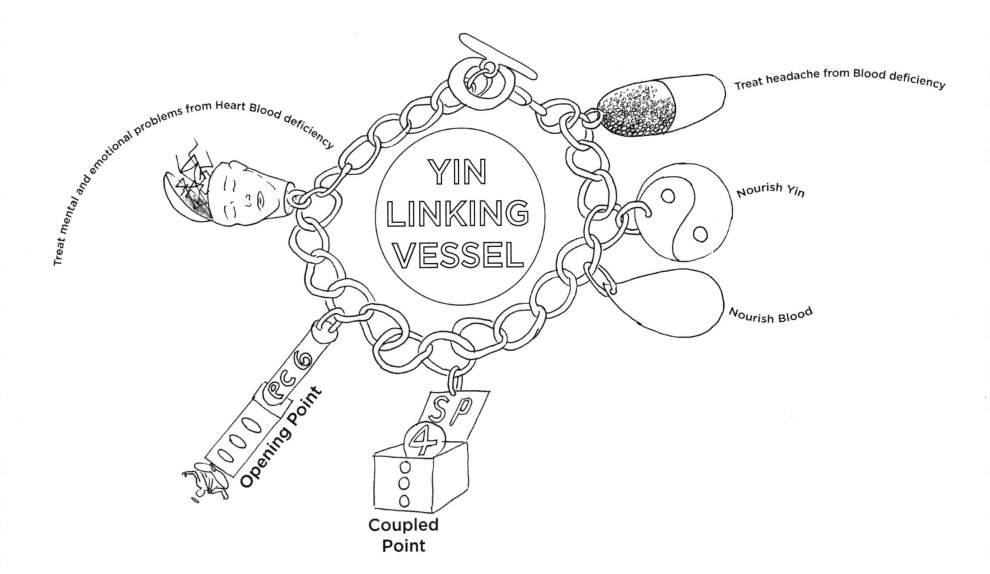

Treat mental and emotional problems from Heart Blood deficiency

Treat headache from Blood deficiency

YIN LINKING VESSEL

Nourish Yin

Nourish Blood

PC 6

Opening Point

SP 4

Coupled Point

Notes

Yang Linking Vessel (Yang Wei Mai)

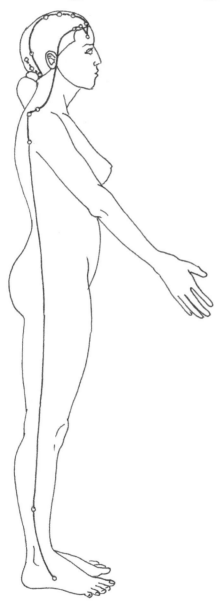

Areas influenced: Lateral aspect of the leg, sides of body, lateral aspect of the neck and head, and ears.

Channels influenced: Triple Burner, Large Intestine, Small Intestine, Stomach, Bladder and Gall Bladder.

CHANNEL FUNCTIONS
TB 5 *Opening Point*
GB 41 *Coupled Point*

- Use in *Shaoyang* fevers

- Influence sides of body

- Affect the ears

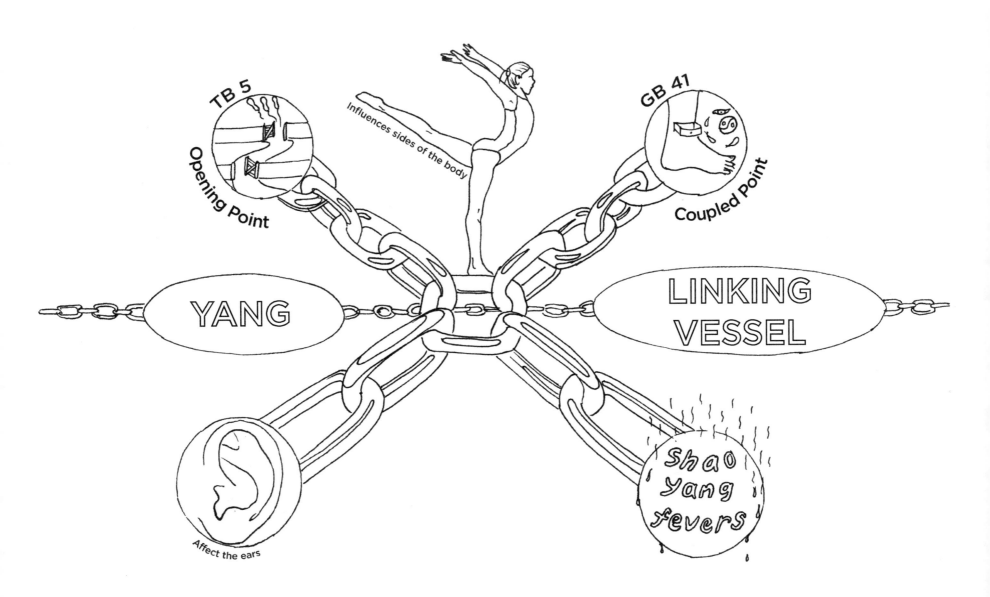

TB 5
Opening Point

Influences sides of the body

GB 41
Coupled Point

YANG

LINKING VESSEL

Affect the ears

Shao yang fevers

Notes